Curbside
Consultation
of the Pancreas

49 Clinical Questions

CURBSIDE CONSULTATION IN GASTROENTEROLOGY
SERIES

SERIES EDITOR, FRANCIS A. FARRAYE, MD, MSc

Curbside Consultation

of the Pancreas

49 Clinical Questions

EDITED BY

Scott Tenner, MD, MPH
Director, Medical Education and Research
Division of Gastroenterology
Maimonides Medical Center
Associate Professor of Medicine
State University of New York—Health Sciences Center
Brooklyn, NY

Alphonso Brown, MD, MS Clin Epi
Co-Director: The Pancreas Center
Assistant Professor of Medicine Harvard Medical School
Division of Gastroenterology, Department of Medicine
The Beth Israel Deaconess Medical Center
Boston, MA

Frank G. Gress, MD
Professor of Medicine
Chief, Division of Gastroenterology and Hepatology
State University of New York
Downstate Medical Center
Brooklyn, NY

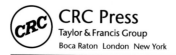

CRC Press
Taylor & Francis Group
Boca Raton London New York

CRC Press is an imprint of the
Taylor & Francis Group, an **informa** business

First published 2010 by SLACK Incorporated

Published 2024 by CRC Press
2385 NW Executive Center Drive, Suite 320, Boca Raton FL 33431

and by CRC Press
4 Park Square, Milton Park, Abingdon, Oxon, OX14 4RN

CRC Press is an imprint of Taylor & Francis Group, LLC

Library of Congress Cataloging-in-Publication Data
Curbside consultation of the pancreas : 49 clinical questions / edited by Scott Tenner, Alphonso Brown, Frank G. Gress.
    p. ; cm. -- (Curbside consultation in gastroenterology)
  Includes bibliographical references and index.
  ISBN 9781556428142 (alk. paper)
  1. Pancreas--Diseases--Miscellanea. I. Tenner, Scott. II. Brown, Alphonso, 1968- III. Gress, Frank G. IV. Series: Curbside consultation in gastroenterology.
  [DNLM: 1. Pancreatitis--diagnosis. 2. Pancreatic Neoplasms--diagnosis. 3. Pancreatic Neoplasms--therapy. 4. Pancreatitis--therapy. WI 805 C975 2010]
  RC857.C87 2010
  616.3'7--dc22
                           2009028005

ISBN: 9781556428142 (pbk)
ISBN: 9781003523765 (ebk)

DOI: 10.1201/9781003523765

Dedication

This book is dedicated to all the students, teachers, and basic and clinical scientists who have committed their lives to the study of pancreatic disease.
It is dedicated to those who care for patients and those who suffer from pancreatic disease. Special thanks to William Steinberg and Peter Banks who have inspired so many to pursue the study of pancreatic disease. Their dedication and commitment to education, research, and excellence in patient care inspired so many physicians and helped so many patients.

—ST

For my family—Deb, Travis, Erin, Morgan, and Abby, whose love, understanding, and patience make it all possible.

—FGG

Contents

Dedication .... *v*

About the Editors .... *xiii*

Contributing Authors .... *xv*

SECTION I: ACUTE PANCREATITIS 1

Question 1   How Much Fluid Should Be Given During the Initial Management of
              Acute Pancreatitis? 3
              Nison Badalov, MD and Scott Tenner, MD, MPH

Question 2   Should I Check a C-Reactive Protein During All Admissions for
              Pancreatitis? 7
              Nison Badalov, MD and Scott Tenner, MD, MPH

Question 3   When Should I Consider Performing a Computed Tomography of the
              Abdomen in Patients With Acute Pancreatitis? 11
              Nison Badalov, MD and Scott Tenner, MD, MPH

Question 4   When Would You Use Antibiotics in Acute Pancreatitis, and Which
              Antibiotics Would You Use? 15
              Nison Badalov, MD and Scott Tenner, MD, MPH

Question 5   What Can Be Done to Minimize Post-Endoscopic Retrograde
              Cholangiopancreatography Pancreatitis? 21
              Nison Badalov, MD and Scott Tenner, MD, MPH

Question 6   What Is the Best Approach to Nutrition in Acute Pancreatitis? 25
              Shishir K. Maithel, MD and Charles M. Vollmer, Jr, MD

Question 7   When Should Gallstones Be Considered the Etiology of Acute
              Pancreatitis? 29
              Nison Badalov, MD and Scott Tenner, MD, MPH

Question 8   When Should an Endoscopic Retrograde Cholangiopancreatography
              Be Performed in Acute Gallstone Pancreatitis? 33
              Nison Badalov, MD and Scott Tenner, MD, MPH

Question 9   My Patient Had a Single Episode of Uncomplicated Gallstone
              Pancreatitis. Should He Have a Cholecystectomy, and, if so, When? 37
              Nison Badalov, MD and Scott Tenner, MD, MPH

Question 10   Should a Cholecystectomy Be Performed on Patients With Acute
              Pancreatitis, No Gallstones, but Sludge in the Gallbladder? 41
              Benjamin E. Young II, MD

Question 11   When Would You Perform Surgery in Acute Pancreatitis? 45
              Nison Badalov, MD and Scott Tenner, MD, MPH

Question 12   What Should Be the Sequence of Investigations for a Patient With
Recurrent, Unexplained Acute Pancreatitis? 49
Nison Badalov, MD and Scott Tenner, MD, MPH

Question 13   How Is Hypertriglyceridemia Treated When Suspected in Causing
Acute Pancreatitis? 55
Susan Ramdhaney, MD and Scott Tenner, MD, MPH

Question 14   My Patient With Crohn's Disease Developed Pancreatitis on Imuran.
Can He Take 6-MP? 59
Nison Badalov, MD and Scott Tenner, MD, MPH

Question 15   My Patient With Acute Pancreatitis Has a Computed Tomography
Scan With Thrombosis of the Splenic Vein. Is It Safe to Anticoagulate
Him? 63
Susan Ramdhaney, MD and Alphonso Brown, MD, MS Clin Epi

SECTION II: CHRONIC PANCREATITIS.. 67

Question 16   How Is the Diagnosis of Chronic Pancreatitis Established? 69
Jonathan Ari Erber, MD and Frank G. Gress, MD

Question 17   What Is the Best Method of Treating Pain in Patients With Chronic
Pancreatitis? 77
Kumaravel Perumalsamy, MD and Scott Tenner, MD, MPH

Question 18   Is There a Role of Pancreatic Enzymes to Treat Pain in Patients With
Chronic Pancreatitis? 83
Sagar Garud, MD, MS and Alphonso Brown, MD, MS Clin Epi

Question 19   What Is the Pathophysiology of Alcohol-Induced Injury
to the Pancreas? 87
Nison Badalov, MD and Scott Tenner, MD, MPH

Question 20   When Should One Suspect Autoimmune Pancreatitis as a Cause of
Acute or Chronic Pancreatitis? 91
Jonathan Ari Erber, MD and William Franklin Erber, MD

Question 21   What Are the Complications of Chronic Pancreatitis? 97
Jonathan Ari Erber, MD and Frank G. Gress, MD

SECTION III: CYSTIC PANCREATIC LESIONS 101

Question 22   My Patient Is a Middle-Aged Woman With an Asymptomatic 5-cm
Fluid-Filled Cyst in the Tail of the Pancreas, Found Incidentally on
Abdominal Computed Tomography Scanning. What to Do Next? 103
Nison Badalov, MD and Scott Tenner, MD, MPH

Question 23   What Is the Best Approach to a Cystic Lesion in the Tail vs Head of the
Pancreas When the Diagnosis Cannot Be Clearly Established? 107
Nison Badalov, MD and Scott Tenner, MD, MPH

Question 24   Endoscopic Ultrasound-Guided Fine Needle Aspiration of a Pancreatic Cyst in This Patient Yielded Fluid With an Amylase of 4500 and a Carcinoembryonic Antigen of 20. Is This Normal? 111
Ilan Aharoni, MD and Scott Tenner, MD, MPH

Question 25   Why Is It Important to Distinguish Serous Cystadenoma and Mucinous Cystadenoma? 115
Hani Abdallah, MD and Alphonso Brown, MD, MS Clin Epi

Question 26   My Hospital Does Not Have an Endoscopic Ultrasonographer. Is It Safe for Me to Use Computed Tomography-Guided Fine Needle Aspiration for a Pancreatic Lesion? 119
Richard O'Farrell, MD

Question 27   How Does One Manage Pseudocysts? 123
Nison Badalov, MD and Scott Tenner, MD, MPH

Question 28   How Do I Determine When a Pseudocyst Has Become Infected? How Do I Manage This? 127
Nison Badalov, MD and Robin Baradarian, MD, FACG

Question 29   My Patient Has a Large Pancreatic Cyst. Should I Involve a Surgeon in the Evaluation and Management of This Situation? 131
John D. Christein, MD

Question 30   When Should Endoscopic Therapy of the Pseudocyst and/or Organized Necrosis in Acute Pancreatitis Be Applied? 135
Nison Badalov, MD and Robin Baradarian, MD, FACG

SECTION IV: PANCREATIC CANCER **141**

Question 31   What Are the Risk Factors for the Development of Pancreatitic Cancer? 143
Nison Badalov, MD and Robin Baradarian, MD, FACG

Question 32   What Is the Best Approach to Staging Pancreatic Cancer? 147
Nison Badalov, MD and Robin Baradarian, MD, FACG

Question 33   What Are the Treatment Options for Early and Locally Advanced Pancreatic Cancer? 153
Paul S. Sepe, MD

SECTION V: OTHER PANCREATIC NEOPLASMS **157**

Question 34   In a Patient With Recurrent Hypoglycemia, How Does One Evaluate for an Insulinoma? 159
Susan Ramdhaney, MD and Alphonso Brown, MD, MS Clin Epi

Question 35   My Patient Has Chronic Diarrhea and Extensive Work-Up Has Been Negative. How to Establish a Diagnosis in a Patient Suspected of Having VIPoma? 163
Jack P. Braha, DO; Robin Baradarian, MD, FACG; and Nison Badalov, MD

Question 36   My Patient Has Reflux Esophagitis in Spite of Daily Omeprazole. His Serum Gastrin on Omeprazole Is 750. What Is the Next Step in Evaluation for Gastrinoma? 167
Susan Truong, HMS III and Alphonso Brown, MD, MS Clin Epi

Question 37   What Masses Mimic Pancreatic Cancer? 171
Susan Truong, HMS III and Alphonso Brown, MD, MS Clin Epi

SECTION VI: BILIARY.......... **175**

Question 38   What Is the Role of Cholangiopancreatoscopy in Pancreaticobiliary Disease? 177
Greg Guthrie, MD and Young Lee, MD

Question 39   My Patient Had a Magnetic Resonance Cholangiopancreatography to Evaluate for Common Bile Duct Stones, but the Reading Includes a "Double Duct Sign." What Does This Mean? Does It Need Endoscopic Retrograde Cholangiopancreatography? 183
Hui Hing (Jack) Tin, MD and Jai Mirchandani, MD

Question 40   How Should I Discuss the Risks of Post-Procedure Pancreatitis With a Patient Whom I Am Consenting for Endoscopic Retrograde Cholangiopancreatography? Do I Really Have to Tell Him He Could Die? 187
Susan Ramdhaney, MD and Alphonso Brown, MD, MS Clin Epi

Question 41   In a Patient With Gallstone Pancreatitis, When Should an Endoscopic Retrograde Cholangiopancreatography and/or Magnetic Resonance Cholangiopancreatography Be Performed Preoperatively? 191
Nison Badalov, MD and Robin Baradarian, MD, FACG

Question 42   I Have a Patient With Suspected Primary Sclerosing Cholangitis. What Do I Need to Know and How Do I Establish the Diagnosis? 197
Ronald Concha-Parra, MD and Frank G. Gress, MD

Question 43   Caroli's Disease, What Do I Need to Know? 203
Mustafa A. Tiewala, MD and Frank G. Gress, MD

Question 44   Choledochal Cyst, What to Do? Watch, Ignore, or Operate? 209
Yuriy Tsirlin, MD and Frank G. Gress, MD

Question 45   What to Do in a Patient Suspected of Having Cholangiocarcinoma? 215
Hui Hing (Jack) Tin, MD and Robin Baradarian, MD, FACG

Question 46   How Often Should I Perform Endoscopic Retrograde Cholangiopancreatography in Order to Retain an Adequate Level of Skill? 221
Susan Ramdhaney, MD and Alphonso Brown, MD, MS Clin Epi

SECTION VII: MISCELLANEOUS..**225**

Question 47   What Is the Best Approach to the Patient With Suspected
Sphincter of Oddi Dysfunction? 227
Nison Badalov, MD and Scott Tenner, MD, MPH

Question 48   When Should a Pancreatic Duct Stent Be Used? 231
Ian Wall, DO and Robin Baradarian, MD, FACG

Question 49   How Do I Evaluate for and Treat Patients With
Autoimmune Pancreatitis? 237
Shishir K. Maithel, MD and Charles M. Vollmer, Jr, MD

Index 241

About the Editors

Scott Tenner, MD, MPH, serves as Director of Medical Education and Research at Maimonides Medical Center, New York. He also serves as an Associate Professor of Medicine at the State University of New York. Dr. Tenner received his doctorate in medicine, his master's in cell biology, and his master's in public health at The George Washington University, Washington, DC. He completed his training in gastroenterology and endoscopy at Brigham and Women's Hospital, Harvard Medical School, Boston. Board certified in both medicine and gastroenterology, he has served as President for the New York Society for Gastrointestinal Endoscopy and currently serves as a Governor and Chair of the National Affairs Committee for the American College of Gastroenterology. Actively involved in teaching and research, Dr. Tenner has authored more than 200 abstracts, papers, chapters, and books. With a focus on diseases of the pancreas, Dr. Tenner is a member of the Research Committee for the American College of Gastroenterology and often serves as a speaker, reviewer, and moderator in subjects of pancreatic disease at national scientific meetings. Despite a busy academic career, Dr. Tenner maintains a busy private practice. He serves as Director of the Brooklyn Gastroenterology and Endoscopy Associates and the Greater New York Endoscopy Surgical Center.

Alphonso Brown, MD, MS Clin Epi, is currently a staff physician at The Beth Israel Deaconess Medical Center, a Harvard teaching hospital. He also holds a teaching appointment at Harvard Medical School. He spends his time between patient care duties and the conduct of translational research.

Frank G. Gress, MD, is Professor of Medicine and Chief, Division of Gastroenterology and Hepatology at the State University of New York (SUNY), College of Medicine and Downstate Medical Center in Brooklyn, NY. Previously, Dr. Gress was Associate Professor of Medicine at Duke University, Durham, NC and served as Clinical Chief for the Gastroenterology Section at the Durham VA Medical Center.

Dr. Gress completed his medical school training at the Mount Sinai School of Medicine in New York, NY; residency in internal medicine at Montefiore Medical Center, Bronx, NY; and his gastroenterology fellowship at the Brooklyn Hospital Center and Methodist Hospital affiliated with SUNY, Health Sciences Center, Brooklyn, NY. After finishing his gastroenterology fellowship, Dr. Gress was awarded the American Society for Gastrointestinal Endoscopy Advanced Endoscopy Scholarship, which was established to support training in advanced therapeutic endoscopy, and he subsequently completed an advanced therapeutic endoscopy fellowship at the Division of Gastroenterology and Hepatology at Indiana University Medical Center in Indianapolis where he trained in the emerging field of endoscopic ultrasound and endoscopic retrograde cholangiopancreatography.

Dr. Gress has published more than 80 articles on original research in highly respected peer-review journals and contributed more than 25 chapters to numerous textbooks on such subjects as clinical gastroenterology, rectal cancer, pancreatitis, pancreatic cancer, advanced endoscopy, training simulators for endoscopy, and the clinical applications of endoscopic ultrasound to name a few. He also lectures regularly at regional and national meetings on these subjects. He also co-authored the textbook *Endoscopic Ultrasonography*, now in its second edition.

Contributing Authors

Hani Abdallah, MD (Question 25)
Assistant Professor of Medicine
Baylor Clinic
Houston, TX

Ilan Aharoni, MD (Question 24)
Osceola Regional Medical Center
Florida Hospital
Kissimmee, FL

Nison Badalov, MD (Questions 1-5, 7-9, 11,
    12, 14, 19, 22, 23, 27, 28, 30-32, 35, 41, 47)
Fellow in Gastroenterology
Maimonides Medical Center
Brooklyn, NY

Robin Baradarian, MD, FACG (Questions 28,
    30-32, 35, 41, 45, 48)
Chief of Gastroenterology
Beth Israel Medical Center
Brooklyn Division
Assistant Professor of Medicine
Albert Einstein School of Medicine
Brooklyn, NY

Jack P. Braha, DO (Question 35)
Gastroenterology Fellow
Maimonides Medical Center
Brooklyn, NY

John D. Christein, MD (Question 29)
Assistant Professor of Surgery
University of Alabama at Birmingham
Birmingham, AL

Ronald Concha-Parra, MD (Question 42)
Gastroenterology Fellow
SUNY Downstate Medical Center
Brooklyn, NY

Jonathan Ari Erber, MD (Questions 16, 20, 21)
Attending Physician
Department of Medicine
Division of Gastroenterology
Maimonides Medical Center
Brooklyn, NY

William Franklin Erber, MD (Question 20)
Attending Physician
Department of Medicine
Division of Gastroenterology
Maimonides Medical Center
Clinical Assistant Professor
SUNY Downstate College of Medicine
Brooklyn, NY

Sagar Garud, MD, MS (Question 18)
PGY-III, Internal Medicine
Beth Israel Deaconess Medical Center
Boston, MA

Greg Guthrie, MD (Question 38)
SUNY Downstate College of Medicine
Brooklyn, NY

Young Lee, MD (Question 38)
Director of Pancreaticobiliary Endoscopy
Brooklyn VAMC
Assistant Professor of Medicine
SUNY Downstate College of Medicine
Brooklyn, NY

Shishir K. Maithel, MD (Questions 6, 49)
Assistant Professor
Division of Surgical Oncology
Emory University
Atlanta, GA

Jai Mirchandani, MD (Question 39)
Assistant Physician
Division of Gastroenterology
Maimonides Medical Center
Brooklyn, NY

Richard O'Farrell, MD (Question 26)
Beth Israel Deaconess Medical Center
Boston, MA

Kumaravel Perumalsamy, MD (Question 17)
High Desert Gastroenterology
Lancaster, CA

Susan Ramdhaney, MD (Questions 13, 15, 34, 40, 46)
Gastroenterology Attending
Brooklyn Gastroenterology and Endoscopy
Brooklyn, NY

Paul S. Sepe, MD (Question 33)
Gastroenterology Fellow
Beth Israel Deaconess Medical Center
Clinical Fellow in Medicine
Harvard Medical School
Boston, MA

Mustafa A. Tiewala, MD (Question 43)
Clinical Assistant Instructor
SUNY Downstate Medical Center
Brooklyn, NY

Hui Hing (Jack) Tin, MD (Questions 39, 45)
Attending in Gastroenterology
Maimonides Medical Center
Brooklyn, NY

Susan Truong, HMS III (Questions 36, 37)
Harvard Medical School
Boston, MA

Yuriy Tsirlin, MD (Question 44)
SUNY Downstate Medical Center
College of Medicine
Brooklyn, NY

Charles M. Vollmer, Jr, MD (Questions 6, 49)
Assistant Professor of Surgery
Beth Israel Deaconess Medical Center
Harvard Medical School
Boston, MA

Ian Wall, DO (Question 48)
Maimonides Medical Center
Brooklyn, NY

Benjamin E. Young II, MD (Question 10)
Resident in Internal Medicine
Beth Israel Deaconess Medical Center
Harvard Medical School
Boston, MA

SECTION I

ACUTE PANCREATITIS

HOW MUCH FLUID SHOULD BE GIVEN DURING THE INITIAL MANAGEMENT OF ACUTE PANCREATITIS?

Nison Badalov, MD and Scott Tenner, MD, MPH

Regardless of etiology, the pathogenesis of acute pancreatitis results in the extravasation of liters of intravascular fluid into the peritoneum. These losses manifest in the development of pancreatic ascites, hypotension, tachycardia, and further destruction of the pancreas, also referred to as pancreatic necrosis. Impairment of the microcirculation of the pancreas appears to lead to pancreatic necrosis. A vicious cycle develops whereby pancreatic inflammation leads to extravasation of protein-rich intravascular fluid into the peritoneum. The intravascular hypovolemia that accompanies acute pancreatitis subsequently leads to a decrease in pancreatic blood flow. Pancreatic ischemia leads to the activation of inflammatory mediators. The decreased blood flow also causes stasis and the development of thrombi leading to subsequent necrosis which then exacerbates the inflammatory process. The association of hemoconcentration, where the hematocrit rises, with pancreatic necrosis illustrates this process (Figure 1-1).

Vigorous intravenous hydration leads to hemodilution and relief of hemoconcentration. This translates into direct benefits for the patient with acute pancreatitis. A decreased hematocrit is associated with mild disease. Also, a falling hematocrit during the first 24 hours of care leads to a decrease in morbidity. Clinical studies with aggressive plasma volume expansion using intravenous dextran to promote hemodilution have suggested efficacy in preventing severe disease. Although dextran is not used clinically at the present time, isotonic saline is our practical alternative. It appears that vigorous intravenous hydration early in the course of acute pancreatitis can prevent the development of necrosis.

Your goal in managing patients with acute pancreatitis is to decrease the hematocrit, hemodilution, blood urea nitrogen, and creatinine and promote renal blood flow. By preventing intravascular depletion of fluid and promoting pancreatic blood flow, pancreatic perfusion is maintained. By maintaining pancreatic perfusion, pancreatic necrosis and the complications of pancreatitis leading to severe disease are prevented (Figure 1-2).

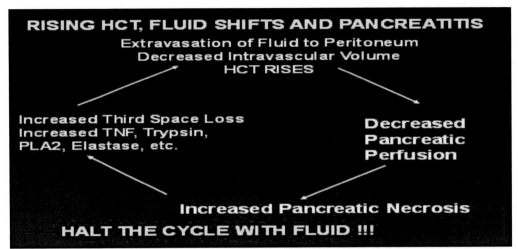

Figure 1-1. In acute pancreatitis, hypoperfusion to the pancreas results in increased pancreatic necrosis, which leads to the release of pro-inflammatory mediators, which in turn exacerbate hypoperfusion, leading to greater necrosis and rise in hematocrit.

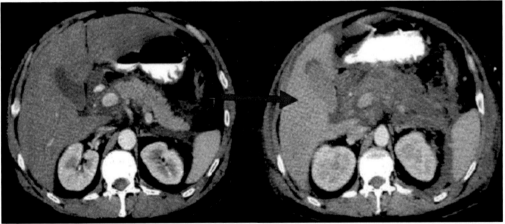

Figure 1-2. Progression to pancreatic necrosis. These images show the progression of pancreatic necrosis in a patient with acute pancreatitis. The dynamic computed tomography scan performed on day 1 shows opacification of the kidneys, spleen, and pancreas. In contrast, a repeat computed tomography scan on day 3 shows opacification of the kidneys and spleen, but no pancreatic opacification. These findings show a loss of pancreatic perfusion between days 1 and 3 of disease. This patient was poorly hydrated (150 cc/hr) and developed acute respiratory distress syndrome, renal failure, and had rise in hematocrit from 42 to 46.

Too often patients with acute pancreatitis are given suboptimal intravenous hydration resulting in pancreatic necrosis and organ failure. How much fluid should be given? Part of the answer is related to the amount of losses the patient presents with and the other part is related to continued losses from the ongoing pancreatic inflammatory process. A patient who presents with hypotension and tachycardia clearly has a need for more aggressive hydration than a patient who presents as normotensive with a normal baseline pulse. Regardless, clinicians must suspect that a patient with acute pancreatitis will subsequently develop serious intravascular fluid losses. One of the markers of severity previously defined by Ranson and colleagues[1] is related to intravascular losses. Ranson and colleagues[1] found that a sequestration (peritoneal pancreatic ascites) of over 6 liters of fluid during the first 48 hours was an independent predictor of severity. A patient with mild disease routinely would lose 3 to 5 liters into the peritoneum.

Not including baseline losses, how much intravenous hydration is needed? If we use the Ranson upper limit of severity 6 liters (expected losses) amount added to the minimal intravenous fluid requirements of a 70-kg person during the first 48 hours (8 liters), intravenous hydration should be at least 300 to 350 cc/hr initially. The rate of hydration is likely to be more important during the first 24 hours where a rising hematocrit has been shown to correlate closely with severe disease. The rate of hydration should be titrated to the hematocrit. The goal is to decrease the hematocrit 5 to 10 points during the first 24 hours.

There are multiple caveats to the basic assumption of the initial rate of hydration. In a patient with acute pancreatitis, in order to guide hydration, the clinician must take into account the age of the patient; underlying cardiac, renal, and pulmonary disease; and the body mass index (BMI) of the patient. Whereas the elderly need to be followed closely, patients with renal disease and cardiovascular disease may need intracardiac monitoring to guide hydration and prevent congestive heart failure. Over the past several years, we have learned that patients who are obese, who have an elevated BMI, are at a higher risk of pancreatic necrosis, organ failure, and death. It is likely that the reason obese patients (those with an elevated BMI) are more likely to have complicated disease is directly related to inadequate intravenous hydration. When one considers that a 100-kg male who is 6 feet, 4 inches needs a baseline of almost 400 cc/hr of hydration, it becomes apparent that if this same patient develops acute pancreatitis, he is far more likely to receive inadequate hydration when compared to a normal person.

Which type of fluid should be used? In order to promote perfusion and maintain intravascular pressure, the fluid should be isotonic. Hypertonic solutions that would maintain or even increase intravascular pressure are being studied, but are considered experimental. The two widely available isotonic solutions are normal saline and Lactated Ringer's.

There are several theoretical benefits to using the more pH-balanced Lactated Ringer's solution for fluid resuscitation compared to normal saline. Although both are crystalloid solutions, the development of non-anion gap hyperchloremic metabolic acidosis associated with the infusion of large volumes of normal saline is well described. Based on the metabolic acidosis associated with large-volume infusion of normal saline and the available evidence suggesting that the inflammation associated with acute pancreatitis is a pH-dependent process, resuscitation with Lactated Ringer's may have significant benefits over normal saline in the early treatment of patients with acute pancreatitis.

Bottom line: in a patient who is otherwise healthy, presenting normotensive with minimal tachydardia, intravenous hydration with Lactated Ringer's at 250 to 350 cc/hr depending on BMI should be initiated and maintained until the acute inflammatory process resolves. The goal is to decrease the hematocrit, at least 3 points from baseline, below 44. Based on animal studies, the goal may be to decrease the hematocrit to the mid 30% range. If the patient presents hypotensive and tachycardic, intravenous hydration should be much more aggressive, 500 cc/hr minimum. Currently, there is no specific therapy available to attenuate the inflammatory response in acute pancreatitis. Instead, practice guidelines universally recommend supportive care with intravenous hydration.

References

1. Ranson JHC, Rifkind RM, Roses DF. Prognostic signs and the role of operative management in acute pancreatitis. *Surgery, Gynecololgy, and Obstetrics*. 1975;139:69.

Bibliography

Baillargeon JD, Orav J, Ramagopal V, Tenner SM, Banks PA. Hemoconcentration as an early risk factor for necrotizing pancreatitis. *Am J Gastroenterol*. 1998;93:2130-2134.

Gardner TB, Vege SS, Pearson RK, Chari ST. Fluid resuscitation in acute pancreatitis. *Clinical Gastroenterology and Hepatology*. 2008;6:1070-1076.

Klar E, Herfarth C, Messmer K. Therapeutic effect of isovolemic hemodilution with dextran 60 on the impairment of pancreatic microcirculation in acute biliary pancreatitis. *Ann Surg*. 1990;211:346-353.

Tenner S. Initial management of acute pancreatitis: critical decisions during the first 72 hours. *Am J Gastroenterol*. 2004;99:2489-2494.

SHOULD I CHECK A C-REACTIVE PROTEIN DURING ALL ADMISSIONS FOR PANCREATITIS?

Nison Badalov, MD and Scott Tenner, MD, MPH

Predicting severity of pancreatitis early in the course of disease is critical to maximize therapy and prevent or minimize organ dysfunction and complications. Unfortunately, the clinician is poor at predicting the severity of acute pancreatitis at the bedside. It has been noted that conservative measures are sufficient for the management of the vast majority of cases of acute pancreatitis; however, the prompt institution of aggressive interventions such as enteral feeding, endoscopic retrograde cholangiopancreatography with sphincterotomy, broad-spectrum antibiotics, and intensive care unit (ICU) monitoring is imperative in specific cases of severe acute pancreatitis in order to decrease morbidity and mortality. Furthermore, delaying ICU admission for more than 24 hours alone has been shown to lead to an increase in mortality. Therefore, it becomes evident that making the distinction between mild and severe cases is of paramount importance, and the sooner this distinction is made, the better.

Unfortunately, the management of patients with acute pancreatitis is complicated by the inability to distinguish mild from severe disease during the early stages. The definition of the severity of acute pancreatitis early in the course of disease (during the first week) is typically based on clinical rather than anatomic parameters. Clinical parameters include organ failure, the development of pancreatic necrosis, and/or scoring systems, such as Ranson and/or APACHE. Laboratory parameters are only on occasion useful. The degree of elevation of serum amylase does not distinguish mild from severe pancreatitis. Although not generally available clinically, levels of interleukin-6, polymorphonuclear leukocyte elastase, phospholipase A2, serum amyloid A, and procalcitonin may prove valuable because their concentrations in blood or urine may serve to separate mild from severe acute pancreatitis. On admission, the creatinine, blood urea nitrogen, and hematocrit may be useful. In addition, a 24-hour hematocrit, 12-hour urinary trypsinogen

---

Table 2-1

C-Reactive Protein for the Determination of Severity of Acute Pancreatitis

Time	Cut-Off Value	Positive Predictive Value	Negative Predictive Value	Accuracy
Admission	>150 mg/dL	59%	79%	75%
24 hours	>150 mg/dL	52%	91%	74%
48 hours	>150 mg/dL	37%	94%	66%
72 hours	>140 mg/dL	86%	79%	83%

---

activation peptide (TAP) levels, and 72-hour C-reactive protein (CRP) may be helpful in distinguishing severe disease. However, further study is needed to establish the role of these markers.

CRP is a simple test that has been used for risk stratification for patients with acute pancreatitis. CRP is an acute phase reactant produced by hepatocytes first described in 1930. It is found in low levels in the bloodstream, and it has been noted to increase soon after an injury, thus serving as a nonspecific marker for inflammatory condition. Several studies have shown a more marked increase in CRP in severe cases of acute pancreatitis compared to mild disease. The marker has been found to predict severe disease with accuracies ranging from 66% to 83%. This variability stems from the use of different cut-off values from as low as 100 mg/dL up to 210 mg/dL as well as measurements performed at different times of the hospital stay (admission to 7 days).

CRP still represents the gold standard with which new potential biologic predictors have to compete. Given its low cost and widespread availability CRP continues to be used. It is an excellent test for distinguishing necrotizing from interstitial (edematous) pancreatitis. The value of CRP is that most patients with necrotizing pancreatitis will have a level over 150 mg/dL at 48 to 72 hours (Table 2-1). Although most patients with pancreatic necrosis will have a more complicated course when compared to patients with interstitial pancreatitis, CRP cannot distinguish patients with mild disease from those with severe disease. Its overall diagnostic accuracy for severe disease is only 70% to 80%. Despite its role in distinguishing necrotizing pancreatitis, CRP is not accurate for predicting infection related to either necrosis or organ failiure. Another limitation to its use in predicting severity of pancreatitis at the onset of presentation or admission is related to the delay in its diagnostic accuracy which typically occurs after 48 to 72 hours. By that time, most patients who will progress will already have obvious signs of severe disease.

For these reasons, CRP is not helpful at admission. Almost all patients with severe disease will have evidence of complications (ie, organ failure) by the time the CRP level rises above 150 mg/dL. The search for an early marker at admission that can help determine severity has been elusive. Further study on TAP is ongoing and may demonstrate TAP as a potential first test to predict severity early in the course of the disease.

In summary, the routine use of CRP as a predictor of severity is not recommended. This is especially true at admission. However, after 48 hours, an elevated CRP is associated with the presence of necrosis. CRP cannot predict infection, organ failure, or outcome of these patients. It remains unclear how an elevated level would alter management, especially given the widespread use and effectiveness of computed tomography for diagnosing necrosis irregardless of the CRP level. Initially, clinical assessment is the only simple and widely available tool that can be used early on to make the distinction between mild and severe acute pancreatitis. Further study is needed before a single marker can be recommended for the determination of severity. The ideal predictor would be a single marker measurable rapidly, reproducibly, and cheaply without discomfort to the patient. CRP is not that marker.

Bibliography

Dambrauskas Z, Bulbinas A, Pundzius Jl, Barauskas G. Value of routine clinical tests in predicting the development of infected pancreatic necrosis in severe acute pancreatitis. *Scand J Gastroenterol.* 2007;42:1256-1264.

Hagiwara A, Miyauchi H, Shimazaki S. Predictors of gastrointestinal complications in severe acute pancreatitis. *Pancreatology.* 2008;8:211-218.

Rettally CA, Skarda S, Garza MA, Schenker S. The usefulness of laboratory tests in the early assessment of severity of acute pancreatitis. *Crit Rev Clin Lab Sci.* 2003;40:117-149.

Schutte K, Malfertheiner P. Markers for predicting severity and progression of acute pancreatitis. *Best Pract Res Clin Gastroenterol.* 2008;22:75-90.

WHEN SHOULD I CONSIDER PERFORMING A COMPUTED TOMOGRAPHY OF THE ABDOMEN IN PATIENTS WITH ACUTE PANCREATITIS?

Nison Badalov, MD and Scott Tenner, MD, MPH

Despite widespread use of computed tomography (CT) of the abdomen in patients with acute pancreatitis, most patients with acute pancreatitis do not need a CT scan. CT scanning is relatively safe, but considerations to radiation exposure and potential nephrotoxicity from contrast are not to be ignored. Earlier concerns that intravenous contrast might affect the course of the disease appear not to be true in humans. There are 4 reasons to order a CT scan in a patient with acute pancreatitis: (1) to clarify the etiology, (2) to determine severity, (3) to evaluate for complications in a patients failing to improve, such as the presence of pancreatic necrosis, and (4) to follow up on anatomical complications of acute pancreatitis, including pseudocysts, necrosis, pseudoaneurysm, etc.

The diagnosis of acute pancreatitis is made by simply finding an elevation of amylase and/or lipase greater than 3 times normal in the setting of clinical symptoms consistent with acute pancreatitis. No imaging such as a CT is needed to make the diagnosis under these conditions. In fact, in this setting an ultrasound of the abdomen is more important to rule out a dilated common bile duct and to evaluate for gallstones. In a patient with equivocal symptoms, and/or an amylase/lipase less than 3 times normal, or a patient in whom the diagnosis is not certain, CT scanning is the best method of determining the etiology. No contrast is needed to simply establish the diagnosis. However, in order to evaluate for necrosis, intravenous contrast is needed.

CT scan is the most important imaging test for excluding other serious intra-abdominal conditions, such as mesenteric infarction or a perforated ulcer; to stage the severity of acute pancreatitis; and to determine whether complications are present, such as involvement of

---

Table 3-1

Computed Tomography Helps Distinguish These Diseases Mimicking Acute Pancreatitis

- Biliary colic/acute cholecystitis
- Perforated hollow viscus
- Mesenteric ischemia or infarction
- Closed-loop intestinal obstruction
- Inferior wall myocardial infarction
- Dissecting aortic aneurysm
- Ectopic pregnancy

---

the gastrointestinal tract or nearby blood vessels and organs, including liver, spleen, and kidney (Table 3-1). Helical CT is the most common technique. If possible, scanning should occur after the patient receives oral contrast, followed by intravenous contrast to identify any areas of pancreatic necrosis. If there is normal perfusion of the pancreas, interstitial pancreatitis is said to be present (Figure 3-1A). Pancreatic necrosis (perfusion defects after intravenous contrast is given) (Figure 3-1B) may not appear until 48 to 72 hours after onset of acute pancreatitis. If infection is suspected, a fine needle aspiration of the pancreatic or peripancreatic bed can be performed.

Contraindications to using intravenous contrast are a patient's history of prior severe allergy (respiratory distress or anaphylaxis) or significant renal impairment (serum creatinine >2 mg/dL). If severe renal impairment requires dialysis, intravenous contrast medium may be used. Hives or less severe allergic reactions with previous administration of iodinated contrast material are not contraindications, but a non-ionic contrast agent should be used, and before the scan 200 mg of hydrocortisone should be administered intravenously every 6 hours for 4 doses and 50 mg of diphenhydramine (Benadryl [McNeil, Fort Washington, PA]) should be given intramuscularly 30 minutes prior to the scan.

It has been suggested that intravenous contrast media early in the course of acute pancreatitis might increase pancreatic necrosis because iodinated contrast medium given at the onset of pancreatitis increases necrosis in experimental rat acute pancreatitis. However, it did not do so in the opossum. Data in humans are conflicting. Two retrospective studies suggested that early contrast-enhanced CT worsened pancreatitis, but this was not corroborated by a third retrospective study.

The severity of acute pancreatitis has been classified into 5 grades (A to E) based upon findings on unenhanced CT (Table 3-2). Grade E pancreatitis represents the most severe disease. At least half of patients with grade E pancreatitis have necrotizing pancreatitis. The majority of patients with pancreatic infection have grade E pancreatitis. This has been further refined into a CT severity index score. The higher the score the more severe the pancreatitis clinically.

Although the presence of gas in the pancreas suggests pancreatic infection with a gas-forming organism, this finding can also accompany sterile necrosis with microperforation of the gut or adjacent pseudocyst into the pancreas. However, the great majority of pancreatic infections occur in the absence of gas on CT scan.

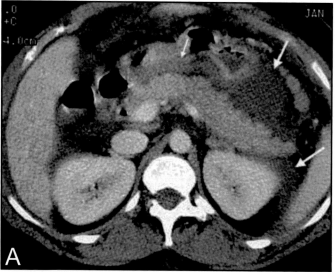

Figure 3-1. Interstitial pancreatitis (A) and necrotizing pancreatitis (B).

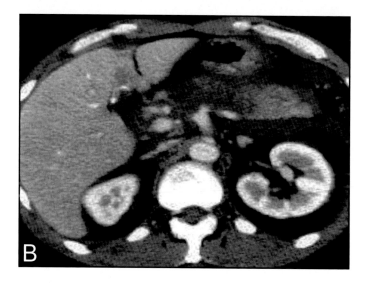

The final role of CT in patients with acute pancreatitis is the need to follow up complications of the disease (eg, pancreatic necrosis, pseudocysts, pseudoaneurysms) that have already been identified. It is not entirely clear how these complications need to be followed. Pseudoaneurysms warrant resection due to the high complication rate. However, it is currently accepted practice that asymptomatic sterile pancreatic necrosis and asymptomatic pseudocysts do not warrant intervention. Therefore, in a patient who is asymptomatic, it is unclear whether further follow-up with CT is needed. However, if pain, weight loss, or fever (sepsis) develops, a follow-up CT is warranted.

Table 3-2

Computed Tomography Grading System of Balthazar

Grade A	Normal pancreas consistent with mild pancreatitis
Grade B	Focal or diffuse enlargement of the gland, including contour irregularities and inhomogeneous attenuation but without peripancreatic inflammation
Grade C	Abnormalities seen in grade B plus peripancreatic inflammation
Grade D	Grade C plus associated single fluid collection
Grade E	Grade C plus two or more peripancreatic fluid collections or gas in the pancreas or retroperitoneum

CT Severity Index Scoring System
1.   Grade A=0, Grade B=1, Grade C=2, Grade D=3, Grade E=4
2.   Absence of necrosis=0, necrosis of up to one-third of the pancreas=2, necrosis of 50%=4, necrosis of >50%=6.

Highest attainable score=10 (Grade E + necrosis >50%)

Bibliography

Balthazar EJ, Ranson JH, Naidich DP, et al. Acute pancreatitis: prognostic value of CT. *Radiology.* 1985;156:767-772.

Balthazar EJ, Robinson DL, Megibow AJ, et al. Acute pancreatitis: value of CT in establishing prognosis. *Radiology.* 1990;174:331.

Uhl W, Roggo A, Kirschstein T, et al. Influence of contrast-enhnaced computed tomography on course and outcome in patients with acute pancreatitis. *Pancreas.* 2002;24:191.

White M, Simeone JF, Wittenberg J. Air within a pancreatic inflammatory mass: not necessarily a sign of abscess. *J Clin Gastroenterol.* 1983;5:173.

QUESTION

WHEN WOULD YOU USE ANTIBIOTICS IN ACUTE PANCREATITIS, AND WHICH ANTIBIOTICS WOULD YOU USE?

Nison Badalov, MD and Scott Tenner, MD, MPH

Antibiotics should always be used when an infection is suspected, until proven otherwise. Patients with acute pancreatitis can develop pneumonia, urosepsis, and other infections that complicate the disease. Chest radiograph and cultures can be taken while antibiotics are given. However, it should be remembered that most patients with acute pancreatitis have fever, tachycardia, and leukocytosis suggesting infection when these findings merely reflect the inflammatory process of pancreatitis. In patients with biliary pancreatitis, who have any signs of biliary sepsis, especially when the bilirubin is elevated suggesting a retained common bile duct stone, broad-spectrum antibiotics should be given. The antibiotic treatment is directed toward the biliary sepsis and not the pancreatitis.

The question of using antibiotics in patients with necrotizing pancreatitis has only recently been clarified. Once sterile pancreatic necrosis exists, prevention of infection is of paramount importance. The presence of infected necrosis typically necessitates surgical debridement. Surgical intervention, while necessary in patients with infected necrosis, increases the morbidity and mortality rate in patients with acute pancreatitis. The surgical management of infected necrosis is an issue that is typically addressed after the first or second week of managing a patient with acute pancreatitis. During the first week, the vast majority of patients with necrosis have sterile necrosis. Surgical intervention during this time is avoided.

The origin of the bacteria leading to pancreatic infection is unclear. Several facts suggest that in acute pancreatitis, there is either direct transmural spread or transmigration of bacteria from the colon. In an attempt to decrease pancreatic infection, initial trials in the 1970s with ampicillin showed a lack of efficacy. Almost 2 decades later, Beger and colleagues[1] showed that only a few antibiotics penetrate pancreatic necrosis, including imipenem, quinolones, and metronidazole. Subsequently, a prospective, randomized trial

comparing imipenem to placebo in the prevention of infected necrosis showed a significant decrease in septic complications. This study was followed by several other trials
demonstrating decreased morbidity and mortality in patients with necrotizing pancreatitis treated with antibiotics within 72 hours of admission. Multiple reviews, including a
Cochrane review[2] in 2004, concluded that pancreatic penetrating antibiotics were useful
in patients with necrotizing pancreatitis. Based on these initial unblinded studies, most
clinicians began the widespread use of antibiotics in patients with necrotizing pancreatitis with the belief that infectious necrosis would be avoided.

Two new, large, multi-center, randomized, double-blinded trials have changed our
opinion regarding the use of antibiotics in sterile necrosis. Isenmann and colleagues[3]
provided evidence that the routine use of ciprofloxacin and metronidazole will not prevent infectious complications in patients with severe pancreatitis. Although this trial was
blinded, there are several limitations to the study. Almost one-third of the patients did
not have surgical or imaging (computed tomography [CT] or magnetic resonance imaging [MRI]) confirmation of the presence of necrosis. Pancreatic necrosis was defined by
an elevated of C-reactive protein. Also, the incidence of infection in the control group
(9%) was unexpectedly low. Of interest, almost half of the placebo patients eventually
were placed on antibiotics on an "open label." As the enrollment of patients in this study
included patients "predicted as having severe disease," this study demonstrates that the
routine use of antibiotics in the absence of pancreatic necrosis is unwarranted.

Dellinger and colleagues[4] performed a multi-center, double-blind, placebo-controlled
randomized study set in 32 centers in North America and Europe. One hundred patients
were equally randomized to 2 groups: meropenem (1 g intravenously every 8 hours) or
placebo within 5 days from the onset of symptoms. The medication was continued for 7 to
21 days. This eloquent study demonstrated no statistically significant difference between
the treatment groups for pancreatic or peripancreatic infection, mortality, or requirement
for surgical intervention. Based on these last 2 studies, in the absence of biliary sepsis
or obvious pancreatic/peripancreatic infection, routine use of antibiotics are not warranted.

Clinically apparent infection of pancreatic necrosis typically occurs after the 10th day
of hospitalization. Infection of the pancreatic necrosis is believed to occur from transloca-
tion of bacteria from the colon. This may help explain why enteral feeding, decreasing
the pathogenic intestinal flora, prevents infection of necrosis. Infection of the pancreatic
necrosis should be suspected when a recurrence of symptoms occur, especially sepsis,
with fever, pain, and leukocytosis. Although patients with sterile necrosis complicated by
organ failure may appear as ill, a "change" in the course occurring between 10 to 14 days
would be consistent with the diagnosis of infected necrosis.

When infection is suspected, the diagnosis is readily established by CT-guided fine
needle aspiration. This procedure is safe and effective in establishing the diagnosis. The
gram stain alone has a sensitivity of almost 95% if carefully examined in a fresh specimen
(Figure 4-1). The procedure is also safe, rarely introducing infection into a sterile field
in the abdomen. If negative, an aspiration can be repeated every 4 to 7 days if infection
continues to be suspected.

In the past, the diagnosis of infected necrosis implied the urgent need for surgical
debridement. This is no longer true. In a persistently ill patient with sepsis and/or organ
failure found to have infected necrosis, surgical debridement should be strongly consid-

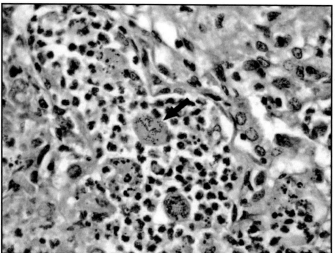

Figure 4-1. Fine needle aspiration was done in a patient who was admitted with necrotizing pancreatitis, with persistent fever, leukocytosis, and worsening renal failure 13 days after admission. Gram stain revealed numerous bacteria (arrow).

ered. However, in a stable patient, with the finding of infected necrosis, maximal supportive care and the use of pancreatic penetrating antibiotics should be provided. It is in these patients, antibiotics such as quinolones, metronidazole, and imipenem should be administered. Although the antibiotics will not likely clear the infection in most patients, the ability to allow time for the formation of a fibrous wall, creating walled-off pancreatic necrosis, will lead to a more minimally invasive approach to draining the pancreatic necrosis.

Recently, Runzi and colleagues[5] studied a series of 28 patients with infected necrosis treated prospectively with antibiotics rather than urgent surgical debridement. In this report, there were 2 deaths among 12 patients who eventually required elective surgical intervention. There were only 2 deaths among 16 patients who were treated with long-term antibiotic therapy. Thus 14 of 16 patients with infected necrosis were successfully treated with no surgical, endoscopic, or radiologic drainage. Further study is needed to clarify which patients with infected necrosis can be treated with antibiotics alone, avoiding debridement and/or drainage of pancreatic necrosis.

In summary, antibiotics should be used when infection is suspected, in the setting of biliary sepsis, in the treatment of infected necrosis. However, based on current evidence, the use of antibiotics in the management of sterile necrosis for the purpose of preventing infection of the necrosis and/or infectious complications is not warranted (Table 4-1).

References

1. Beger HG, Bittner R, Block S, et al. Bacterial contamination of pancreatic necrosis: a prospective clinical study. *Gastroenterology.* 1986;91:433.
2. Bassi C, Larvin M, Villatoro E. Antibiotic therapy for prophylaxis against infection of pancreatic necrosis in acute pancreatitis. *Cochrane Database Syst Rev.* 2003;4:CD002941.
3. Isenmann R, Runzi M, Kron M, et al. Prophylactic antibiotic treatment in patients with predicted severe acute pancreatitis: a placebo controlled, double blind trial. *Gastroenterology.* 2004;126:997-1004.
4. Dellinger EP, Tellado JM, Soto NE, et al. Early antibiotic treatment for severe acute necrotizing pancreatitis: randomized, double blind, placebo controlled study. *Ann Surg.* 2007;245(5):674-683.
5. Runzi M, Niebel W, Goebell H, et al. Severe acute pancreatitis: nonsurgical treatment of infected necroses. *Pancreas.* 2005;30:195-199.

Table 4-1

Randomized Placebo-Controlled Studies Evaluating Intravenous Antibiotic Prophylaxis of Acute Necrotizing Pancreatitis

Study Reference	Antibiotic Dose	N		Pancreatic Infection		Sepsis		Mortality	
		Antibiotic	Placebo	Antibiotic	Placebo	Antibiotic	Placebo	Antibiotic	Placebo
Pederzoli	Imipenem (500 mg tid)	41	33	5	10	6	16	3	4
Saino	Cefuroxime (1.5 g tid)	30	30	9	12	11	13	1	7
Schwarz	Ofloxacin (200 mg bid) Metronidazole (500 mg qid)	13	13	8	7	4	6	0	2
Delcenserie	Ceftazidime (2 g q 8 h) Amikacin (7.5 mg/kg q 12 h) Metronidazole (0.5 g q 8 h)	11	12	0	7	NA	NA	1	3
Nordback	Imipenem (500 mg tid)	25	33	2	14	7	25	2	5
Isenmann	Ciprofloxacin (400 mg bid) Metronidazole (500 mg bid)	58	56	5	3	13	14	3	4
Dellinger	Meropenem (1 g q 8 h)	50	50	9	6	16	24	10	9

Bibliography

Dickerson RN, Vehe KL, Mullen Beger HG, Bittner R, Block S, Buchler M. Bacterial contamination of pancreatic necrosis: a prospective study. *Gastroenterology.* 1986;91:433-438.

Pederzoli P, Bassi C, Vesentini S, Campedelli A. A randomized multicenter trial of antibiotic prophylaxis of septic complications in acute necrotizing pancreatitis with imipenem. *Surg Obstet Gynecol.* 1993;176:480-483.

WHAT CAN BE DONE TO MINIMIZE POST-ENDOSCOPIC RETROGRADE CHOLANGIOPANCREATOGRAPHY PANCREATITIS?

Nison Badalov, MD and Scott Tenner, MD, MPH

Identification of the risk factors for post-endoscopic retrograde cholangiopancreatography (ERCP) pancreatitis is essential to recognize high-risk cases in which ERCP should be avoided if possible, or in which protective endoscopic or pharmacologic interventions should be considered. If a patient has 1 or more risk factors, avoidance of ERCP should be strongly considered. Diagnostic ERCP has largely been replaced by magnetic resonance cholangiopancreatography (MRCP) and endoscopic ultrasound (EUS), which should be considered first-line in patients in whom the ERCP is merely for diagnostic purposes. Risk factors for developing post-ERCP pancreatitis have been assessed in various studies and include patient-, procedure-, and operator-related factors (Table 5-1).

On reviewing the literature, the general consensus of the patient-related factors include: young age, female gender, suspected sphincter of Oddi dysfunction (SOD), recurrent pancreatitis, prior history of post-ERCP pancreatitis, and patients with normal bilirubin. The procedure-related factors include: pancreatic duct injection, difficult cannulation, pancreatic sphincterotomy, pre-cut access, and balloon dilatation. The operator or technical factors are controversial. Although a high-volume endoscopist should intuitively have lower rates, studies in general do not show this to be true. However, trainee (fellows) participation has been shown to be a significant risk factor for the development of post-ERCP pancreatitis.

In general, the more likely a patient is to have an abnormal common bile duct and/or pancreatitic duct, the less likely the patient will develop post-ERCP pancreatitis. The role of patient factors, including age, suspicion of SOD, and prior history of post-ERCP

Table 5-1

Factors Increasing the Risk of Post-Endoscopic Retrograde Cholangiopancreatography Pancreatitis

Choosing the Wrong Patient: Patient-Related Factors
Young age, female gender, suspected sphincter of Oddi dysfunction, recurrent pancreatitis, prior history of post-ERCP pancreatitis, patients with normal bilirubin.

Choosing the Wrong Procedure: Procedure-Related Factors
Pancreatic duct injection, difficult cannulation, pancreatic sphincterotomy, pre-cut access, and balloon dilatation.

Choosing the Wrong Endoscopist: Operator/Technical-Related Factors
Although a high-volume endoscopist should intuitively have lower rates, studies in general do not show this to be true. However, trainee (fellows) participation has been shown to be a significant risk factor for the development of post-ERCP pancreatitis.

---

pancreatitis, and technical factors, including number of pancreatic duct injections, minor papilla SOD, operator experience, and involvement of a trainee/fellow have all been shown to increase the risk of post-ERCP pancreatitis.

The patient who is most at risk of developing post-ERCP pancreatitis is a female with suspected choledocholithiasis and a normal bilirubin, who undergoes a sphincterotomy and no stone is found or who is suspected of having SOD and undergoes biliary and pancreatic manometry. In this patient population, more than one-quarter or one-third of patients develop post-ERCP pancreatitis, respectively. MRCP and EUS, which do not cause pancreatitis, can provide useful information (perhaps as accurate as ERCP) in many of these cases and are preferred modalities in the initial evaluation of ruling out choledocholithiasis.

Multiple medications have been studied to prevent post-ERCP pancreatitis, including nifedipine, nitroglycerin, nonsteroidal anti-inflammatory drugs (NSAIDs), steroids, somatostatin, octreotide, etc. Although there has been great interest in developing medications that can prevent post-ERCP pancreatitis, studies have failed to identify a medication worthy of widespread use.

Pancreatic stent placement clearly decreases the risk of post-ERCP pancreatitis in high-risk patients (Figure 5-1). Placement of pancreatic duct stents has become a standard practice for patients who are thought to be at risk for pancreatitis after the procedure. Pancreatic duct stent placement is effective presumably by preventing cannulation-induced edema that can cause pancreatic duct obstruction. Pancreatic sphincter hypertension is believed to be an important causative factor in post-ERCP pancreatitis and may explain the high risk of pancreatitis in patients with SOD. There is prolonged alleviation of ductal obstruction when pancreatic stents are placed. Typically, 3 to 5 French unflanged pancreatic stents are used in the following settings: SOD, difficult cannulation, biliary orifice balloon dilatation, and pre-cut sphincterotomy. Thirteen trials—6 prospective randomized controlled trials and 7 case control studies—have been published evaluating the role of pancreatic

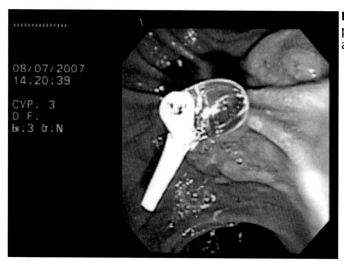

Figure 5-1. Pancreatic duct stent preventing severe acute pancreatitis in high-risk patients.

stent placement in the prevention of post-ERCP pancreatitis. When combined, all reported studies cumulatively included a total of 1500 high-risk patients undergoing ERCP; only 1 patient developed severe pancreatitis after a pancreatic duct stent had been placed. In a large retrospective review of 2283 patients with a total of 2447 ERCPs, 3 French unflanged stents were more effective in reducing the incidence of post-ERCP pancreatitis (p=0.0043), more likely to pass spontaneously (p=0.0001), and less likely to cause ductal changes (24% vs 80%) when compared to larger 4, 5, or 6 French stents. Aside from the obvious benefits in preventing post-ERCP pancreatitis regarding morbidity and mortality, prophylactic stent placement is a cost-effective strategy for the prevention of post-ERCP pancreatitis for high-risk patients.

Guidewire cannulation, whereby the biliary and/or pancreatic duct are initially cannulated by a guidewire inserted through the catheter or sphincterotome, has been shown to decrease the risk of pancreatitis. By avoiding cannulation with contrast agents, thus minimizing the risk of hydrostatic injury to the pancreas, the incidence of acute pancreatitis appears to be dramatically decreased. In a study of 400 consecutive patients who underwent ERCP by a single endoscopist, randomized to initial cannulation with contrast vs initial cannulation by guidewire under fluoroscopic control, pancreatitis rates were profoundly different. No cases of acute pancreatitis were seen in the guidewire group compared to 8 cases in the standard contrast group (p<0.001). Cannulation success rates between the standard contrast and guidewire techniques were comparable 98.5% vs 97.5%.

In summary, multiple studies have shown that patient-related factors are as important as technical factors in predicting the risk of acute pancreatitis following ERCP. Risk stratification will allow endoscopists to better identify patients who are at risk. ERCP should be avoided in patients with a low likelihood of pathology (stones, strictures, masses) as complications appear to be inversely proportional. Multiple studies have failed to adequately identify a drug that consistently prevents post-ERCP pancreatitis in all patients. However, until effective, safe, and low cost prophylactic drugs are identified and made available, selective use in high-risk groups may be warranted. The best strategy for prevention of post-ERCP pancreatitis appears to be selecting patients carefully and avoiding the procedure in those patients who it will have very little benefit, and using guidewire cannulation and judicious placement of pancreatic duct stents in high-risk patients.

Bibliography

Cheng CL, Risk factors for post ERCP pancreatitis: a prospective multicenter study. *Am J Gastroenterol.* 2006;101:139-147.

Freeman ML, DiSario JA, Nelson DB, et al. Risk factors for post-ERCP pancreatitis: a prospective, multicenter study. *Gastrointest Endosc.* 2001;54:425-434.

Freeman ML, Guda NM. Prevention of post-ERCP pancreatitis: a comprehensive review. *Gastrointest Endosc.* 2004;59:845-864.

Mehta SN, Pavone E, Barkun JS, et al. Predictors of post-ERCP complications in patients with suspected choledo-cholithiasis. *Endoscopy.* 1998;30:457-463.

WHAT IS THE BEST APPROACH TO NUTRITION IN ACUTE PANCREATITIS?

Shishir K. Maithel, MD and Charles M. Vollmer, Jr, MD

The role of nutrition in acute pancreatitis continues to evolve. The dogma in treating acute pancreatitis has been to restrict oral intake in order to "rest the pancreas." However, withholding nutrition entirely from these patients is not appropriate primarily because the systemic inflammatory response in acute pancreatitis leads to a catabolic state. Adequate supply of nutrients plays an important role in the recovery of these patients. The early use of total parenteral nutrition (TPN) in patients with acute pancreatitis has not been shown to be beneficial and should generally be avoided due to increased infectious complications, greater morbidity, and trends to greater mortality in patients given TPN when compared to control patients.

If the pancreatitis is deemed mild, special nutritional feedings are not required. Intravenous hydration is adequate until the patient is no longer having significant abdominal pain, tenderness, nausea, or vomiting, at which point oral feedings can be initiated (usually days). The question of which factors can predict those patients who will respond poorly to re-feeding has been addressed. When patients with acute pancreatitis were fed 250 kcal/day at the clinician's discretion, 21% developed pain on re-feeding and their hospital stay was nearly doubled (33 vs 18 days). A lipase level that was greater than 3-fold elevated the risk of a pain relapse after re-feeding (39% vs 16%). Conversely, most patients with lower lipase levels prior to re-feeding did not develop pain. However, lipase can remain elevated for prolonged periods of time after pancreatitis and it seems reasonable to offer clear liquids with no (or very few) calories when pain and nausea have subsided regardless of the enzyme levels. If tolerated, gradual advancement to regular food can ensue.

Can patients be fed soon after admission, even while the pain persists and amylase remains elevated? The doctrine has been that oral feeding should be withheld in patients with acute pancreatitis early in the course to prevent continued stimulation of pancreatic exocrine function. Experimental studies in humans have suggested this not to be true, and that, in fact, the pancreas in patients with acute pancreatitis is in a state of inactivity that cannot be stimulated. One group of investigators found early re-feeding to be safe, and early institution of an oral diet decreased the length of stay. However, a recent meta-analysis which included three studies on early re-feeding in patients with mild acute pancreatitis found an increase in pain relapses. If re-feeding is attempted, there does not appear to be a difference if a low-fat diet is used compared to a clear liquid diet as the initial meal. If re-feeding fails, controversy exists regarding the optimal route of achieving nutrition. Some feel enteral feeding is superior physiologically to TPN, yet the access tubes required are poorly tolerated for the long-term periods required (often weeks) and therefore TPN may provide better quality of life for these patients, despite the heightened risk of infection.

In patients with severe acute pancreatitis, the role of enteral feeding is more important and more clearly established. The immunologic response that starts with the systemic inflammatory response syndrome can lead to early multiple organ dysfunction syndrome (MODS). Patients who do not develop early MODS can manifest a compensatory anti-inflammatory response syndrome which suppresses immunity and predisposes to sepsis, thereby increasing the risk of late MODS, and ultimately, death. Furthermore, patients with pancreatic necrosis are generally not able to physically ingest food for long periods of time, often 3 to 4 weeks, as inflammation simmers and remodeling occurs. After multiple studies found that enteral nutrition will reduce septic morbidity in conditions such as trauma and thermal injury, its role in severe acute pancreatitis was studied. The initial thinking was that early enteral nutrition would maintain the integrity and function of the intestinal barrier while providing adequate nutrition. More specifically, bypassing the stomach and duodenum using a nasojejunal tube should also decrease stimulation of the pancreas, in theory.

In patients with acute pancreatitis, the use of enteral nutrition has traditionally been delayed by the old belief that pancreatic rest is required to prevent complications. This reasoning appears untrue. To date, a series of randomized trials comparing enteral vs parenteral nutrition have been performed in patients with severe acute pancreatitis. These studies in general show a decrease in morbidity and mortality (in one study) in patients given enteral nutrition early in the course of disease. These benefits are maximized when enteral feeds are started early (<72 hours) and at least 50% to 60% of goal calories are delivered. Enteral nutrition has also proven more cost effective than parenteral nutrition, which has been estimated to cost approximately 4 times that of enteral nutrition when delivering equal calories. By providing nutrients and altering the bacterial flora, there is a significant decrease in the development of infected pancreatic necrosis. Stable computed tomography scan scores of pancreatitis severity in both enterally and parenterally fed patients show that distal (post-ligament of Treitz) feeding does not worsen severity by stimulating pancreatic exocrine function. The immune modulating and overall benefits of early enteral feeding in severe pancreatitis have been demonstrated using various parameters. Enterally fed patients show significant reductions in levels of C-reactive protein and oxidant stress. There is a consensus among the trials demonstrating decreased infectious complications, length of stay, and significant cost savings. These patients also tend to spend less time in the intensive care unit (ICU) and have a lower incidence of sepsis, MODS, the need for operative intervention, and mortality when compared with their parenterally fed counterparts.

Post-ligament of Treitz enteral feeding is clearly beneficial in critically ill patients with severe pancreatitis, barring any prohibitive intestinal obstruction or functional ileus. However, nutrition support technology has trailed the need for quick, safe, and effective feeding in complex critically ill patients. Aside from open surgery, which is not a good option in these patients, distal enteral access can be gained fluoroscopically, percutaneously, or endoscopically. Endoscopic placement expedites appropriate enteral access in critically ill patients, reduces the risks of patient transport associated with alternative approaches, and relies on direct visual guidance to minimize risk of complications, including duodenal perforation and transcolonic placement, two rare but potentially devastating complications of radiographically placed jejunal feeding tubes. One method involves using an ultraslim video endoscope to place a double lumen gastric aspiration, jejunal feeding tube (DLFT) beyond the ligament of Treitz. The endoscopic route also provides additional diagnostic information of potential benefit to patients. Endoscopic placement of post-ligament of Treitz feeding tubes has the potential to facilitate the delivery of early enteral nutrition and improve the care of critically ill patients with severe acute pancreatitis.

Although the nasojejunal route has been used in several trials, a nasogastric route may also be safe. A UK group (Eatock et al) randomized 50 patients with severe pancreatitis to nasogastric vs nasoenteric tube feedings. No difference was seen in the ability to tolerate feedings, in markers of inflammation or in morbidity or mortality between the groups. This prospective study comparing nasogastric to nasojejunal feeding found no differences in the length of hospital stay or complications in patients with severe acute pancreatitis. Current data do not demonstrate a significant difference in aspiration when comparing gastric and post-pyloric feeding tubes. Post-ligament of Treitz feeding in these patients, however, does not eliminate the universally feared risk of pulmonary aspiration, a complication that can be from antegrade (from oropharyngeal secretions) as well as retrograde etiology. To date, there is no definitive way to prevent aspiration in critically ill ICU patients. Many strategies have been suggested to minimize the risk, including oral decontamination with antiseptics, avoiding the supine position, use of small caliber feeding tubes, keeping the head of bed above 45 degrees, and proper nursing education. The use of gastric residual volumes to determine tolerance of gastric feeding is poorly standardized and does not correlate well with the incidence of aspiration. The correct rate of infusion is also a topic of much discussion. Large randomized studies are needed to determine if jejunal feeding is actually superior to gastric feeds, but these have thus far been difficult to achieve on account of limited patient accrual.

Further study is needed regarding initiation of enteral nutrition in acute pancreatitis. In general, patients with mild disease can be fed as tolerated earlier than previously believed. TPN plays a role in those patients who suffer a more protracted clinical course (moderate pancreatitis). In patients with severe disease, where a nothing-by-mouth status will likely last for more than 3 days (eg, patients with necrosis, on a ventilator), early enteral feeding is the preferred method. In this age of cost-effective health care delivery, early enteral nutrition has the added advantage of providing the greatest benefit to these patients with optimal clinical outcomes and cost efficiency.

Bibliography

Abou-Assi S, Craig K, O'Keefe SJ. Hypocaloric jejunal feeding is better than total parenteral nutrition in acute pancreatitis: results of a randomized comparative study. *Am J Gastroenterol.* 2002;97:2255-2262.

Eatock FC, Chong P, et al. A randomized study of early nasogastric vs. nasojejunal feeding in severe acute pancreatitis. *Am J Gastroenterol.* 2005;100:432-439.

Eckerwall GE, Axelsson JB, Andersson RG. Early nasogastric feeding in predicted severe acute pancreatitis: a clinical, randomized study. *Ann Surg.* 2006;244:959-965.

Jacobson B, Vander A, Viliet MA, et al. A prospective randomized trial of clear liquids vs low fat solid diet as the initial meal in mild acute pancreatitis. *Clinical Gastroenterology and Hepatology.* 2007;5:946-951.

McClave SA, Greene LM, Snider HL, et al. Comparison of the safety of early enteral vs parenteral nutrition in mild acute pancreatitis. *JPEN J Parenter Enteral Nutr.* 1997;21(1):14-20.

McClave SA, Marsano LS, Lukan JK. Enteral access for nutritional support: rationale for utilization. *J Clin Gastroenterol.* 2002;35(3):209-213.

O'Keefe SJD, Foody W, Gill S. Transnasal endoscopic placement of feeding tubes in the ICU. *JPEN J Parenter Enteral Nutr.* 2003;27(5):349-354.

Olah A, Pardavi G, Belagyi T, et al. Early nasojejunal feeding in acute pancreatitis is associated with a lower complication rate. *Nutrition.* 2002;18(3):259-262.

Petrov MS, van Santvoort HC, Besselink MGH. Oral refeeding after onset of acute pancreatitis: a review of literature. *Am J Gastroenterol.* 2007;102:2079-2084.

Windsor ACJ, Kanwar S, Li AGK, et al. Compared with parenteral nutrition, enteral feeding attenuates the acute phase response and improves disease severity in acute pancreatitis. *Gut.* 1998;42:431-435.

When Should Gallstones Be Considered the Etiology of Acute Pancreatitis?

Nison Badalov, MD and Scott Tenner, MD, MPH

Gallstones are the most common cause of acute pancreatitis (Figure 7-1). The pathogenesis of gallstone pancreatitis depends on the presence of a common bile duct (CBD) stone. The vast majority of these stones pass easily and quickly. In some patients, choledocholithiasis or gallstones in the CBD may lead to severe disease complicated by biliary sepsis. Defining the presence of a persistent CBD stone as the cause of severe, complicated acute pancreatitis can be problematic. Although considered the gold standard for cholelithiasis, abdominal ultrasonography in the setting of acute pancreatitis is not sensitive for the evaluation of choledocholithiasis. Gallstones may be present in the CBD even in the absence of biliary ductal dilatation on abdominal ultrasound.

Laboratory testing may assist in the early identification of gallstone pancreatitis and/or CBD stones. Although elevated transaminases have a poor sensitivity for determining gallstone pancreatitis, a high specificity can be reached with laboratory testing. A greater than 3-fold elevation of aspartate aminotransferase (AST) or alanine aminotransferase (ALT) in the presence of acute pancreatitis has a positive predictive value of 95% in diagnosing gallstones as the etiology of pancreatitis.[1] However, it must be stressed that almost half of all patients with gallstone pancreatitis will have normal liver function tests.

Most stones pass readily from the CBD. However, in a small percentage of patients, the stones persist in the CBD and may need to be removed at endoscopic retrograde cholangiopancreatography (ERCP). On multivariate analysis, serum total bilirubin on hospital day 2 was the best predictor of a persistent CBD stone. A serum total bilirubin level greater than 1.35 mg/dL has a sensitivity of over 90%. Unfortunately, the specificity for CBD stones is only 63%. Other investigators have found that a rising bilirubin or transaminases within 24 to 48 hours of admission for acute pancreatitis predicted a persistent CBD stone.

Figure 7-1. Ultrasound image showing gallstones in the gall-bladder in a patient with acute pancreatitis. Notice the classic hyperechoic stone in the gall-bladder and shadowing that follows from the transducer.

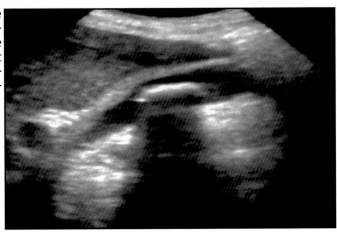

In patients with idiopathic acute pancreatitis, gallstones are the most common cause. The patient with idiopathic pancreatitis is one who has a normal ultrasound of the abdomen, no history of alcoholism, normal serum triglyceride level, and no obvious offending medications. In this patient, the gallstone likely passes or was too small (microlithiasis, biliary sludge) to be seen by normal imaging. Microlithiasis (Figure 7-2) is widely agreed upon as the most common cause of idiopathic acute recurrent pancreatitis (IARP). Although technically different, the terms microlithiasis (stones <3 mm) and biliary sludge (suspension of crystals and mucin) are often used interchangeably. It is unclear if microlithiasis/sludge causes acute pancreatitis or simply denotes the likelihood that a stone was present that passed. Studies on the prevalence of microlithiasis in patients with IARP vary from 7% to 75%. To even make the issue more complicated, repeated exposure to microlithiasis may lead to papillary stenosis and sphincter of Oddi dysfunction. The optimum method of detecting microlithiasis is yet to be established. Transabdominal ultrasound, the most commonly used method, is only 50% sensitive. Endoscopic ultrasound is more sensitive approaching 75% to 80%. Repeat evaluations may increase the yield. Duodenal aspirates have 66% sensitivity and ERCP has a sensitivity of 85%. Cholecystokinin (CCK [Sincalide, Bristol-Myers Squibb, New York, NY]) can be given prior to the procedure to increase the yield to 95%. Once an aspirate is obtained, the collected bile needs to be centrifuged at 2000 rpm for 10 minutes and examined on polarized microscopy. Therapy for microlithiasis can significantly reduce the risk of recurrent pancreatitis. Several options exist though laparoscopic cholecystectomy is preferred. ERCP with sphincterotomy and oral treatment with ursodeoxycholic acid (Urso [Axcan Pharma, Birmingham, AL] or Actigall [Novartis, Basel, Switzerland]) can be used alternatively. If oral therapy is used, long-term use is necessary. No randomized, blinded trials exist to establish efficacy.

In summary, gallstones should be suspected as the cause of acute pancreatitis all the time. Gallstones are the most common cause of acute pancreatitis. Gallstones are almost always the cause when the transaminases are greater than 3 times normal. Gallstones are the most common cause when the etiology is not clear (eg, in idiopathic pancreatitis). Prior to blaming other etiologies, gallstones should be ruled out, especially since this is the most common cause and readily treatable to prevent recurrence (eg, cholecystectomy).

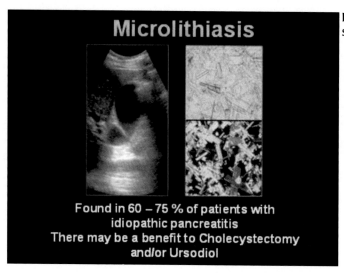

Figure 7-2. Microlithiasis: ultrasound and microscopic images.

References

1. Tenner S, Dubner H, Steinberg W. Predicting gallstone pancreatitis with laboratory parameters: a meta-analysis. *Am J Gastroenterol.* 1994;89:1863-1869.

Bibliography

Chang L, Lo SK, Stabile BE, Lewis R, de Virgilio C. Gallstone pancreatitis: a prospective study on the incidence of cholangitis an clinical predictors of retained common bile duct stones. *Am J Gastroenterol.* 1998;93:527-531.

Cohen ME, Slezak L, Wells CK, Andersen DK, Topazian M. Prediction of bile duct stones and complications in gallstone pancreatitis using early laboratory trends. *Am J Gastroenterol.* 2001;96:3305-3311.

Steinberg WM, Chari ST, Forsmark CE, et al. Management of acute idiopathic recurrent pancreatitis. *Pancreas.* 2003;27:103-117.

When Should an Endoscopic Retrograde Cholangiopancreatography Be Performed in Acute Gallstone Pancreatitis?

Nison Badalov, MD and Scott Tenner, MD, MPH

The pathogenesis of gallstone pancreatitis depends on the presence of a common bile duct (CBD) stone. The vast majority of these stones pass easily and quickly. In some patients, gallstones can persist in the CBD and may lead to severe disease complicated by biliary sepsis. Defining the presence of a persistent CBD stone as the cause of severe, complicated acute pancreatitis can be problematic. Although considered the gold standard for cholelithiasis, abdominal ultrasonography in the setting of acute pancreatitis is not sensitive for the evaluation of choledocholithiasis and CBD stones. Gallstones may be present in the CBD even in the absence of biliary ductal dilatation on abdominal ultrasound.

Laboratory testing may assist in the early identification of CBD stones. Although elevated transaminases have a poor sensitivity for determining gallstone pancreatitis, a high specificity can be reached with laboratory testing. A greater than 3-fold elevation of aspartate aminotransferase (AST) or alanine aminotransferase (ALT) in the presence of acute pancreatitis has a positive predictive value of 95% in diagnosing gallstones as the etiology of pancreatitis.[1] However, most stones pass the CBD regardless of elevation of transaminases. On multivariate analysis, serum total bilirubin on hospital day 2 was the best predictor of a persistent CBD stone. A serum total bilirubin level greater than 1.35 mg/dL has a sensitivity of over 90%. Unfortunately, the specificity for CBD stones is only 63%. Other investigators have found that a rising bilirubin or rising transaminases within 24 to 48 hours of admission for acute pancreatitis predicted a persistent CBD stone.

Table 8-1
Randomized Trials Comparing Urgent Endoscopic Retrograde Cholangiopancreatography to Medical Therapy

Study	Number of Patients	Time of ERCP*	Outcome
Neoptolemos	121	72 hours	Decreased morbidity in severe disease
Fan	195	24 hours	Decrease in biliary sepsis
Folsch	121	72 hours	No effect on outcome excluded bilirubin >5 mg/dL

*ERCP was performed within a time frame prior to the hours cited.

Regardless of findings on laboratory testing and ultrasonography, endoscopic retrograde cholangiopancreatography (ERCP) remains the gold standard in identifying whether gallstones are retained in the CBD. Unfortunately, depending on the patient, there is a 5% to 10% risk of developing pancreatitis if ERCP is performed. Endoscopic ultrasound (EUS) and magnetic resonance imaging (MRI) provide excellent visualization of the CBD and can be used to determine the presence of CBD stones with less risk.

The role of ERCP in acute pancreatitis continues to evolve (Table 8-1). Since the days of Opie, Osler, and Halstead, clinicians have pondered the following question: will removing a stone impacted at the ampulla affect the course of acute pancreatitis? It must be remembered that the vast majority of stones that cause acute pancreatitis rapidly pass out of the CBD. Three published studies addressing the issue of urgent ERCP in the management of patients with acute pancreatitis build upon each other and provide clarity. The first randomized study by Neoptolemos and colleagues[2] found that early ERCP (within 72 hours) decreased morbidity in patients with severe acute pancreatitis (defined by Ranson's criteria). No benefit of ERCP in patients with acute pancreatitis was seen in patients with mild disease. Similarly, Fan and colleagues[3] showed that early ERCP in patients with acute pancreatitis (within 24 hours) decreased the incidence of biliary sepsis in patients with severe acute pancreatitis significantly, 12% vs 0%. However, there were no differences between the two groups regarding local or systemic complications of acute pancreatitis. Interestingly, the incidence of complications was lower in Fan's series compared to that of Neoptolemos. This suggests that earlier intervention, within 24 hours, may be more beneficial than waiting 72 hours.

The role of ERCP in patients with severe acute pancreatitis was further clarified in a final study by Folsch and colleagues.[4] In this study, patients with obvious biliary obstruction, bilirubin greater than 5 mg/dL, were excluded. Unlike the earlier studies by Neoptolemos and Fan, by excluding jaundiced patients, this study showed that early ERCP was no more effective than medical treatment in patients with acute pancreatitis.

Thus, early ERCP, within 24 to 72 hours, is effective in patients with severe acute pancreatitis who have evidence of biliary obstruction, cholangitis, and an elevated bilirubin. There is no evidence that urgent ERCP alters the course of patients with severe acute pancreatitis in the absence of biliary obstruction.

References

1. Tenner S, Dubner H, Steinberg W. Predicting gallstone pancreatitis with laboratory parameters: a meta-analysis. *Am J Gastroenterol.* 1994;89:1863-1869.
2. Neoptolemos JP, London NJ, James D, Carr-Locke DL. Controlled trail of urgent endoscopic retrograde cholangiopancreatography and endoscopic sphincterotomy versus conservative management for acute pancreatitis due to gallstones. *Lancet.* 1988;3:979-983.
3. Fan ST, Lai EC, Mok FP, et al. Early treatment of acute biliary pancreatitis by endoscopic papillotomy. *N Engl J Med.* 1993;328:228-232.
4. Folsch UR, Nitsche R, Ludtke R, et al. Early ERCP and papillotomy compared with conservative treatment for acute biliary pancreatitis. *N Engl J Med.* 1997;336:237-242.

My Patient Had a Single Episode of Uncomplicated Gallstone Pancreatitis. Should He Have a Cholecystectomy, and, if so, When?

Nison Badalov, MD and Scott Tenner, MD, MPH

Calculous biliary disease remains the leading cause of acute pancreatitis. Gallstones should be considered the cause of acute pancreatitis in any patient who has stones identified on imaging of the gallbladder following an attack of acute pancreatitis. This is true even if the patient has a significant history of alcohol use, hypertriglyceridemia, and/or an obvious offending medication. Although an elevated aspartate aminotransferase (AST) and/or alanine aminotransferase (ALT) greater than 3 times normal is associated with gallstones as the cause with a specificity of 95%, the sensitivity is too low to predict accuracy. Almost half the patients with gallstone-induced acute pancreatitis have normal transaminases.

The pathophysiology of gallstone pancreatitis is not entirely clear. Transient obstruction of the pancreatic duct by a gallstone in the common bile duct (CBD) was first attributed as the cause by Opie at the turn of century. The Opie theory or "common channel" theory describes the reflux of duodenal juice into the pancreatic duct secondary to transient sphincter of Oddi dysfunction after stone passage or ductal hypertension secondary to sudden pancreatic duct obstruction. It remains unclear if the pressure or the presence of bile itself causes the acute pancreatitis.

Although most stones that cause acute pancreatitis readily pass from the CBD into the duodenum, some remain in the CBD and require either endoscopic retrograde cholangiopancreatography (ERCP) or surgical removal. Regardless of the fate of the initial CBD stone that caused the initial attack of acute pancreatitis, there is a risk that a recurrent attack will occur if the gallbladder remains.

Figure 9-1. This is the computed tomography (CT) of a 45-year-old gentleman who had been admitted for acute pancreatitis, mild disease. The initial CT showed interstitial pancreatitis, normal perfusion of the pancreas. One month after discharge, failing to follow up for a cholecystectomy for the known gallstones, the patient was readmitted with a more complex course. Note on this second CT, the pancreas previously normal, now with necrosis of the head and body. The gallstone in the gallbladder is also noted. This image drives home the point to perform early cholecystectomy to prevent a recurrent attack.

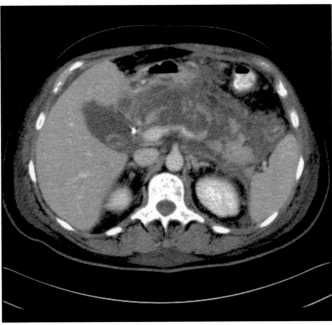

Due to a combination of stasis and lithogenic bile, a gallbladder that produces gallstones will continue to develop gallstones even if the stone passes or is removed. Thus, it is a standard of care that in a patient with complications from gallstones, a cholecystectomy be performed to prevent future complications.

Laparoscopic cholecystectomy allows early surgery that is feasible and safe but often technically difficult in patients with gallstone pancreatitis compared to uncomplicated cholelithiasis. Multiple series have shown almost no mortality and no significant morbidity. Most deaths are in elderly patients with co-morbid disease.

Thus, cholecystectomy is usually performed following an episode of gallstone pancreatitis to prevent recurrent disease. Current management of gallstone pancreatitis is laparoscopic cholecystectomy with or without intraoperative cholangiography (if CBD stone is suspected intraoperatively). If stones are identified in the CBD, ERCP with endoscopic sphincterotomy and stone removal can be performed intraoperatively or postoperatively. Preoperative ERCP is reserved for patients with evidence of concomitant cholangitis, persistently abnormal liver enzymes (after exclusion of other common causes), and choledocholithiasis seen or suspected on imaging.

The timing of surgery has been debated. Early surgery has the potential disadvantage of operating on a sick patient and increased difficulty of dissection due to inflammation in the region of the gallbladder may occur. Alternatively, delayed surgery places the patient at risk of recurrent pancreatitis or other complications of cholelithiasis or choledocholithiasis (Figure 9-1). The timing of cholecystectomy is based not only on the physician preference but on the severity of pancreatitis. In the era of open cholecystectomy, Kelly and Wagner[1] demonstrated that surgery for severe biliary pancreatitis (more than 3 Ranson's criteria) was best delayed until resolution of the inflammatory process, but delaying operative intervention in mild to moderate cases was unnecessary. Despite this, the surgical literature has a preferred early resection of the gallbladder in patients with mild disease.

In cases of mild pancreatitis, United Kingdom guidelines for the management of acute pancreatitis recommend definitive treatment of gallstones, ideally within 2 weeks and no longer than 4 weeks. In reality, cholecystectomy is often delayed. Delay in cholecystectomy has been associated with a high unplanned re-admission rate due to recurrent cholecystectomy. It appears that patients with mild to moderate gallstone pancreatitis can safely undergo early laparoscopic cholecystectomy without waiting for normalization of laboratory values or resolution of symptoms. The incidence of recurrent pancreatitis following gallstone pancreatitis has been evaluated by multiple authors. Burch and colleagues[2] looked at 102 patients who were discharged after recovery and scheduled for elective surgery. Of the 102 patients, 37 (36%) were lost to follow-up, refused further treatment, or were operated on elsewhere. Of the 65 patients who remained in their care after discharge, 29 (44%) suffered recurrent pancreatitis (35%) or biliary tract disease (9%) before elective surgery. Most of these recurrences (66%) occurred within 3 months and 2 occurred within 1 week.

In summary, although delay in surgery remains the standard of care for severe gallstone pancreatitis, the timing of cholecystectomy for mild to moderate pancreatitis leans to early laparoscopic removal, preferably prior to discharge from the hospital. The fear is that a delay in surgery will lead to recurrent pancreatitis, a more severe attack, or possibly even death from a preventable etiology.

References

1. Kelly TR, Wagner DS. Gallstone pancreatitis: a prospective randomized trial of the timing of surgery. *Surgery.* 1988;104:600-605.
2. Burch JM, Feliciano DV, Matox KL, Jordon GL. Gallstone pancreatitis: the question of time. *Arch Surg.* 1990;125:853-860.

Bibliography

Cameron DR, Goodman AJ. Delayed cholecystectomy for gallstone pancreatitis: re-admissions and outcomes. *Ann R Coll Surg Engl.* 2004;86:358-362.

Rosing DK, de Virgilo C, Yaghoubian A, et al. Early cholecystectomy for mild to moderate gallstone pancreatitis shortens hospital stay. *J Am Coll Surg.* 2007;205:762-766.

Sanjay P, Yeeting S, Whigham C, et al. Endoscopic sphincterotomy and interval cholecystectomy are reasonable alternatives to index cholecystectomy in severe acute gallstone pancreatitis. *Surg Endosc.* 2008;22:1832-1837.

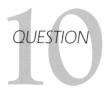
SHOULD A CHOLECYSTECTOMY BE PERFORMED ON PATIENTS WITH ACUTE PANCREATITIS, NO GALLSTONES, BUT SLUDGE IN THE GALLBLADDER?

Benjamin E. Young II, MD

Microlithiasis has been defined as tiny stones (1 to 2 mm) that are missed on imaging studies. In contrast, biliary sludge is a mixture of microscopic matter in the gallbladder, commonly including cholesterol crystals, glycoproteins, mucin, cellular debris, and calcium salts. In practice, since biliary sludge may contain microlithiasis, these two terms have been used interchangeably. In addition, radiologists often use both terms for the same description. As the clinical outcome of patients with biliary sludge and microlithiasis appears to be the same, as of now, it is not unreasonable to lump both terms together.

In patients with intact gallbladders, it has been estimated that up to 60% to 80% of acute idiopathic pancreatitis may be due to microlithiasis. Prior to evaluating or treating a patient for acute pancreatitis suspected of being caused by microlithiasis, other causes should be ruled out. The patient should be diagnosed as having acute idiopathic pancreatitis. Thus there should be a negative transabdominal ultrasound, no history of alcoholism, normal triglycerides, and no obvious offending medication. In these patients, no clear consensus has been reached, however, diagnostic and therapeutic options exist.

Evidence supports treating microlithiasis if identified on imaging (Table 10-1). First is empiric cholecystectomy. This is still commonly practiced and is not unreasonable. Alternatively, duodenal aspirate of bile after cholecystokinin (CCK [Sincalide, Bristol-Myers Squibb, New York, NY]) stimulation can be utilized for diagnostic confirmation. The sensitivity of this procedure is 66%. The procedure requires at least a couple of cc's of bile, a centrifuge, and a phase contrast microscope. Direct common bile duct aspiration during endoscopic retrograde cholangiopancreatography (ERCP) has been performed

Table 10-1

Outcome of Treatment of Microlithiasis in the Prevention of Recurrent Pancreatitis

	Ros and Colleagues	*Lee and Colleagues*
Recurrences if untreated	12/18 (67%)	8/11 (73%)
Recurrences if treated	3/19 (16%)	1/10 (10%)
Follow-up	42 to 44 months	Not provided

and may increase the sensitivity. Endoscopic ultrasound (EUS) has become a popular alternative for further diagnostic testing due to its higher sensitivity for microlithiasis and sludge (Figure 10-1).[1] EUS also has the advantage of evaluating several alternative causes for acute idiopathic pancreatitis, including pancreas divisum, neoplasms, and undiagnosed chronic pancreatitis.

There is a reasonable amount of literature suggesting that intervention for recurrent idiopathic pancreatitis is warranted. One study by Saraswat and colleagues[2] looked at a total of 23 patients with recurrent idiopathic acute pancreatitis or unexplained biliary pain, both groups having abnormal biliary sludge (defined as a single cholesterol mono-hydrate crystal or >25 calcium bilirubinate granules/slide on microscopic examination). These 23 patients underwent either cholecystectomy (n=2) or sphincterotomy (n=21) and remained asymptomatic for a mean follow-up period of 23 months. This was in comparison to the 1 patient who refused either intervention and over a 12-month period continued to experience pain at the same frequency as prior to the study. Another study by Lee and colleagues[3] showed that patients with idiopathic pancreatitis who were found to have biliary sludge and subsequently received either cholecystectomy or papillotomy had fewer recurrences up to 7 years in follow-up. In addition to cholecystectomy for recurrent idiopathic pancreatitis thought to be related to biliary sludge/microlithiasis, Ros and colleagues[1] showed that oral ursodeoxycholic acid may be effective.

Despite these and other studies that show a clear benefit to intervening, there does not seem to be a consensus on the means of intervention. In a series in *Pancreas* appropriately titled "Controversies in Clinical Pancreatology," members of the American Pancreatic Association had varying responses to a clinical scenario of a patient with recurrent, seemingly idiopathic pancreatitis.[4] While some of the members advocated either cholecystectomy or sphincterotomy, many actually supported biliary drainage. Points of contention included the sensitivity of biliary drainage for the diagnosis of microlithiasis, estimated to be anywhere from 49% to 82%, the error rate of diagnosis and subsequent unnecessary cholecystectomies, as well as the importance of a step-wise, diagnostic approach involving ERCP to not only sample the bile, but rule out pancreatic structural abnormalities and perform sphincter of Oddi manometry. In the absence of studies focusing on direct comparison of different methods, a consensus agreement has not been reached.

In summary, although no consensus exists, cholecystectomy, oral ursodeoxycholic acid, or biliary drainage appear to be a reasonable option for patients with idiopathic

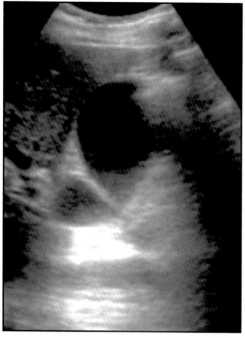

Figure 10-1. Transabdominal ultrasound image showing sludge in the gallbladder.

acute pancreatitis. However, the evidence weighs heavily on the presence of microlithiasis/sludge. Based on the limited data available, a conservative approach with serial transabdominal ultrasound may be the best approach with watchful waiting until US shows true gallstones.

References

1. Ros E, Navarro S, Bru C, Garcia-Puges A, Valderrama R. Occult microlithiasis in idiopathic acute pancreatitis: prevention of relapses by cholecystectomy or ursodeoxycholic acid therapy. *Gastroenterology*. 1991;101:1701-1709.
2. Saraswat VA, Sharma BC, Agarwal DK, Kumar R, Negi TS, Tandon RK. Biliary microlithiasis in patients with idiopathic acute pancreatitis and unexplained biliary pain: response to therapy. *J Gastroenterol Hepatol*. 2004;19(10):1206-1211.
3. Lee SP, Nicholls JF, Park HZ. Biliary sludge as a cause of acute pancreatitis. *N Engl J Med*. 1992;326(9):589-593.
4. Steinberg WM, Barkin J, Bradley EL III, DiMagno E, Layer P. Recurrent "idiopathic" acute pancreatitis: should a laparoscopic cholecystectomy be the first procedure of choice? *Pancreas*. 1996;13(4):329-334.

WHEN WOULD YOU PERFORM SURGERY IN ACUTE PANCREATITIS?

Nison Badalov, MD and Scott Tenner, MD, MPH

The most common role of the surgeon is 2-fold in acute pancreatitis: (1) to remove the gallbladder in cases of gallstone pancreatitis to prevent recurrent disease and (2) to debride pancreatic necrosis or drain a pancreatic abscess should these complications develop. Whereas all patients with gallstone pancreatitis will need a cholecystectomy, most patients with acute pancreatitis will have a mild course and not need surgical intervention. Most patients with complicated disease, even in the presence of pancreatic pseudocysts or necrosis, will also not require surgical intervention.

In patients with gallstone pancreatitis, a cholecystectomy is needed to prevent recurrent disease. Studies have clearly shown that in a patient who develops acute pancreatitis and has a gallbladder with gallstones, a recurrent attack will occur in as many as 50% in 3 months if the gallbladder is not removed. A consensus conference of surgical guidelines suggested that in mild and severe gallstone pancreatitis, cholecystectomy should be performed as soon as the patient has recovered and the inflammatory process has subsided, typically prior to discharge.

With regard to pancreatic necrosectomy, the data are more complicated and evolving. Studies in the 1980s suggested that early necrosectomy (within the first week of hospitalization for severe disease) improved mortality. However, in the only randomized study comparing early (within 72 hours of admission) vs late necrosectomy (>12 days after admission) the mortality of early operation was greater than later debridement (56% vs 27%). Some investigators have reported that it is important to differentiate sterile necrosis from infected necrosis by fine needle aspiration of the pancreas. Sterile necrosis can be managed nonoperatively as the mortality of this condition without surgery is less than 5%.

Figure 11-1. Computed tomography-guided fine needle aspiration of the pancreas, or peripancreatic bed, is a safe and accurate method of determining infection of pancreatic necrosis.

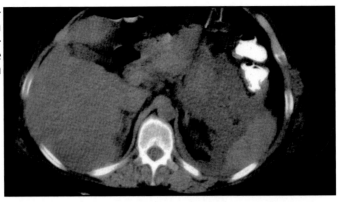

Figure 11-2. Pancreatic necrosis appears isodense to liquid and often "tricks" clinicians in assuming that a liquid is present. Unfortunately, necrotizing pancreatitis is a solid as shown in this figure. Drainage by endoscopy or radiologic catheter placement is not effective, often leading to worsening infection. Surgical debridement is needed as the method of choice to remove the necrosis.

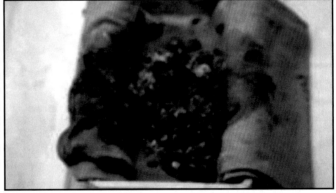

Infected necrosis (as documented by fine needle aspiration of the pancreas), on the other hand, has been historically regarded as an indication for surgical debridement because of the belief that infected necrosis treated medically has a nearly uniform fatal outcome (Figure 11-1). This has led to the recommendation that patients who are not improving on maximal medical therapy or who show new signs of organ failure should have a fine needle aspiration of the pancreas. The finding of infection should then lead to a consideration of surgical intervention. Pancreatic necrosis is solid and cannot be drained by a catheter (Figure 11-2).

On the other hand, surgical therapy of infected pancreatic necrosis carries a substantial mortality of 15% to 73%, especially when it is carried out early within the first few weeks of the disease. Thus, it is unclear if the higher mortality rates that have been reported with infected necrosis are merely the result of the underlying disease or the early surgical intervention. It has been shown that delay in surgical debridement beyond the second week in patients with pancreatic necrosis is associated with a lower mortality rate. However, in a patient with gas-producing organisms (Figure 11-3), or whom multisystem organ failure is progressing, surgical intervention early may be needed.

The concept that infected pancreatic necrosis requires prompt surgical debridement has been challenged by several reports of patients who have been treated by antibiotic therapy alone. Recently, a large series of 28 patients with infected necrosis treated prospectively with antibiotics rather than urgent surgical debridement.[1] In this report, there

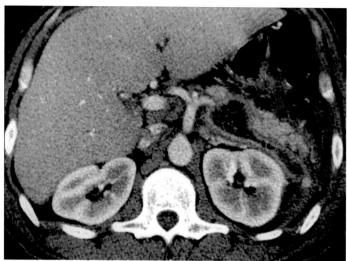

Figure 11-3. This is the computed tomography of a 66-year-old gentleman who presented with acute pancreatitis and within 4 days, multisystem organ failure developed. The patient was found to have gas in the body of the pancreas. Surgical resection revealed a "gangrenous necrotic pancreas." Failure to perform an urgent necrosectomy in such patients, though a rare finding, will result in death.

were 2 deaths among 12 patients who eventually required elective surgical intervention. There were only 2 deaths among 16 patients who were treated with long-term antibiotic therapy. Thus 14 of 16 patients with infected necrosis were successfully treated with no surgical, endoscopic, or radiologic drainage.

The types of surgery that have generally been recommended have included necrosectomy with closed continuous irrigation via indwelling catheters, necrosectomy and open packing, or necrosectomy with closed drainage without irrigation. There have not been randomized prospective trials comparing these procedures. All are generally considered to provide equal benefit in skilled surgical centers. More recently, several additional procedures have been introduced that are less invasive than standard open surgical debridement of infected necrosis. These techniques have generally been reserved for patients with infected pancreatic necrosis who are too ill to undergo prompt surgical debridement (such as those with organ failure and/or serious co-morbid disease), including laparoscopic necrosectomy with placement of large caliber drains under direct surgical inspection and percutaneous catheter drainage of infected necrosis. Other minimally invasive approaches, including endoscopic or a combined endoscopic and laparoscopic approach, may become more commonly used as skill and technology advance. The role of nonsurgical therapy for infected necrosis needs to be compared to endoscopic therapy in controlled trials.

Even in the absence of infected pancreatic necrosis, there is a concept that removing necrotic tissue in severe sterile necrosis may overcome organ failure. Clinicians must be cautious as patients with sterile necrosis may appear quite ill, with fever, leukocytosis, and organ failure. The desire to simply remove necrotic tissue in an attempt to control organ failure must be tempered against the fact that most patients with sterile necrosis will do well with a conservative approach. Minimally invasive surgery within the first 2 to 3 weeks of severe sterile necrosis has not been compared prospectively with the continuation of medical therapy and thus far is an evolving technology.

In summary, surgical intervention in acute pancreatitis is reserved to a small subset of patients (Table 11-1). Patients with gallstone pancreatitis and who have gallstones in their pancreas should undergo cholecystectomy at the time of discharge. Failure to

---

Table 11-1

Surgery Indications in Acute Pancreatitis

Gallstone pancreatitis and gallstones in gallbladder
Sterile necrosis—worsening organ failure
Infected necrosis
- Early if sepsis fails to resolve with antibiotics
- Progression of multisystem organ failure
- Gas-producing organisms in pancreas
- Infected pseudocyst, abscess—unable to perform endoscopic/radiologic drainage
- Presence of a pseudoaneurysm

---

perform a cholecystectomy early may increase the risk of a recurrent attack. In patients with infected necrosis, surgical debridement will likely be necessary. However, by providing intense intravenous antibiotics, a delay in surgery will likely allow a minimally invasive approach. In patients who have pancreatic necrosis, whether infected or sterile, who develop multisystem organ failure, necrosectomy may be needed early.

Bibliography

Adler DG, Chari ST, Dahl TJ, et al. Conservative management of infected necrosis complicating severe acute pancreatitis. *Am J Gastroenterol.* 2003;98:98-103.

Baril NB, Ralls PW, Wren SM, et al. Does an infected peripancreatic fluid collection or abscess mandate operation? *Ann Surg.* 2000;231:361-367.

Fernandez-del Castillo C, Rattner DW, Makary MA, et al. Debridement and closed packing for the treatment of necrotizing pancreatitis. *Ann Surg.* 1998;228:676-684.

Runzi M, Niebel W, Goebell H, et al. Severe acute pancreatitis: nonsurgical treatment of infected necroses. *Pancreas.* 2005;30:195-199.

WHAT SHOULD BE THE SEQUENCE OF INVESTIGATIONS FOR A PATIENT WITH RECURRENT, UNEXPLAINED ACUTE PANCREATITIS?

Nison Badalov, MD and Scott Tenner, MD, MPH

Acute recurrent pancreatitis (ARP) results most commonly from alcohol abuse or gallstone disease. Less common causes that must be excluded include tumors, triglycerides, and obvious offending medications. If initial evaluation fails to detect the cause of ARP, the diagnosis of idiopathic acute recurrent pancreatitis (IARP) is given. This diagnosis is made in 10% to 30% of patients with acute pancreatitis. Evaluation and therapy is important because in more than 50% of patients with IARP, recurrent episodes may lead to chronic pancreatitis.

The initial evaluation includes a search for evidence of alcohol abuse, drug-induced pancreatitis, and a family history of pancreatitis. A history of weight loss suggests underlying chronic pancreatitis or a malignancy. Laboratory analysis may be helpful. Pancreatitis resulting from gallstones, microlithiasis, or drugs is more often associated with a greater elevation of amylase than lipase. The amylase level as compared to lipase tends to be lower in alcoholic pancreatitis. The ratio of lipase to amylase may help distinguish alcoholic from nonalcoholic pancreatitis, with an increased ratio suggesting alcohol-induced disease. Elevations of the transaminases, aspartate aminotransferase (AST) and/or alanine aminotransferase (ALT), in the setting of acute pancreatitis suggest the presence of gallstones as the etiology. A serum ALT greater than 3 times normal in the setting of acute pancreatitis has a 95% positive predictive value for gallstone pancreatitis. Metabolic causes of pancreatitis should be excluded by checking the serum calcium and triglyceride levels. These values should be measured soon after admission or well after resolution of pancreatitis. It should be noted that serum calcium and triglycerides can

---

Table 12-1

Prior to Establishing the Diagnosis of Idiopathic Pancreatitis

- Evaluate for alcohol abuse (>3 drinks a day for >5 years)
- Ultrasound gallbladder to rule out gallstones
- Consider magnetic resonance cholangiopancreatography
- If aspartate and/or alanine aminotransferase >3 times normal, gallstone pancreatitis likely
- Obtain serum calcium and triglyceride level (repeat in 4 weeks if elevated but not high enough)
- Computed tomography with intravenous contrast to rule out tumor
- Rule out Class 1 or Class 2 drugs (Badalov system)

---

decrease during the hospitalization of acute pancreatitis and borderline results should be rechecked 2 to 4 weeks after discharge.

Transabdominal ultrasound is a simple, inexpensive, and highly sensitive procedure for evaluating the biliary tract. Computed tomography (CT) more accurately delineates the pancreas and may also help identify a cause. Although some investigators have recommended performing CT only when the first attack is severe, when the course is complicated, or in the elderly, it is the opinion of most pancreatologists that patients with no clear etiology should undergo a CT scan even on the first episode.

The extent of evaluation required before conferring the diagnosis of IARP varies among studies. The purist would demand a complete and exhaustive work-up before the diagnosis. However, most investigators would use this diagnosis when the more limited evaluation described above fails to reveal an etiology. After ruling out the more common diagnoses listed in Table 12-1, a more extensive evaluation should be considered. The remainder of this review focuses on establishing a diagnosis for relatively rare causes of acute pancreatitis.

Microlithiasis (Biliary Sludge)

This is widely agreed upon as the most common cause of IARP. Although technically different, the terms *microlithiasis* (stones <3 mm) and *biliary sludge* (suspension of crystals and mucin) are often used interchangeably. It is unclear if microlithiasis/sludge causes acute pancreatitis or simply denotes the likelihood that a stone was present that passed. Studies on the prevalence of microlithiasis in patients with IARP vary from 7% to 75%. To even make the issue more complicated, repeated exposure to microlithiasis may lead to papillary stenosis and sphincter of Oddi dysfunction (SOD). The optimum method of detecting microlithiasis is yet to be established. Transabdominal ultrasound, the most commonly used method, is only 50% sensitive. Endoscopic ultrasound (EUS) is more sensitive approaching 75% to 80%. Repeat evaluations may increase the yield. Duodenal aspirates have a 66% sensitivity. Endoscopic retrograde cholangiopancreatography (ERCP) has a sensitivity of 85%. Cholecystokinin (CCK [Sincalide, Bristol-Myers Squibb, New York, NY]) can be given prior to the procedure to increase the yield to 95%.

Table 12-2
Sphincter of Oddi Dysfunction Classification

Biliary Type	*Pancreatic Type*
Type I	
Biliary-type pain	Pancreatic-type pain
Elevated liver function tests	Elevated amylase/lipase
Common bile duct dilatation	Pancreatic duct dilatation
Delayed drainage	Delayed drainage
Type II	
Biliary-type pain + 1 above feature	Pancreatic-type pain + 1 above feature
Type III	
Biliary-type pain	Pancreatic-type pain

Once an aspirate is obtained, the collected bile needs to be centrifuged at 2000 rpm for 10 minutes and examined on polarized microscopy. Therapy for microlithiasis can significantly reduce the risk of recurrent pancreatitis. Several options exist though laparoscopic cholecystectomy is preferred. ERCP with sphincterotomy and oral treatment with ursodeoxycholic acid (Urso [Axcan Pharma, Birmingham, AL] or Actigall [Novartis, Basel, Switzerland]) can be used alternatively. If oral therapy is used, long-term use is necessary. No randomized, blinded trials exist to establish efficacy.

Sphincter of Oddi Dysfunction

Although many experts, particularly advanced endoscopists, believe that SOD is a major cause of IARP, overzealous endoscopists performing ERCP may have unfortunately created more harm than benefit. Regardless, SOD is a frequent and treatable cause of IARP and is seen in roughly one-third of these patients. Patients with SOD are classified as having either biliary or pancreatic SOD. Table 12-2 shows the classification system widely accepted for categorizing such patients as described by Hogan and Geenen.[1]

Sphincter of Oddi manometry (SOM) is the gold standard for diagnosing SOD. The procedure employs a water-perfused catheter system, inserted endoscopically into the common bile duct or pancreatic duct to measure pressure. The diagnosis is established by finding a hypertensive sphincter pressure greater than 40 mm Hg. However, the exact normal vs pathologic pressure has not been well studied. In patients with type I disease, treatment without a measurement is reasonable. However, in patients with types II and III SOD, SOM should be considered mandatory. Endoscopic spincterotomy is the therapy of choice and is believed to decrease the risk of recurrent pancreatitis by reducing sphincter pressure. Placement of a stent to decrease the risk of post-ERCP pancreatitis is indicated in patients with type III (and possibly type II disease). No randomized, blinded trials exist to establish efficacy.

Pancreas Divisum

Pancreas divisum, where the main pancreatic duct (Wirsung) embryologically fails to join the dorsal duct of Santorini, is the most common congential malformation of the pancreas and gastrointestinal tract, affecting 5% to 8% of the population. Although controversial, many investigators, especially advanced endoscopists, believe that pancreas divisum is a common cause of IARP. Both magnetic resonance cholangiopancreatography (MRCP) and ERCP can establish the diagnosis. In select experts, the diagnosis can be established by EUS. Treatment is directed toward relief of outflow obstruction from the minor papilla which, in patients with pancreas divisum, drains the majority of the pancreas. Endoscopic and surgical therapies decrease the rate of recurrent pancreatitis by 70% to 90% in select series. No randomized, blinded trials exist to establish efficacy.

Genetic Factors

Although the past decade has resulted in a better understanding of genetic factors involved in acute pancreatitis, especially hereditary pancreatitis, the prevalence of genetic factors in IARP remains unclear. More important, the discovery of the genetic factors in patients with IARP does not necessarily mean any therapeutic benefits.

Hereditary pancreatitis is a rare disorder of autosomal dominant transmission caused by a mutation in cationic trypsinogen. The disorder is not affected by gender, becomes clinically apparent by the teens, but can be delayed to the mid 30s. In patients with acute pancreatitis before the age of 20, evaluation is necessary. Most patients will have a family history of acute or chronic pancreatitis or pancreatic cancer. The diagnosis can be made by genetic analysis. Establishing the diagnosis assists in family planning and screening for pancreatic cancer but rarely helps patients with IARP.

Cystic fibrosis is the most common genetic disease affecting the exocrine pancreas. It is passed by recessive mutations in the cystic fibrosis transmembrane conductance regulator (CFTR) transport protein. Most patients with cystic fibrosis develop pancreatic insufficiency and malabsorption due to diminished pancreatic bicarbonate and enzyme secretion. Acute recurrent or chronic pancreatitis develops in only 2% of patients and interestingly does not show the other phenotypic presentations of the disease. This is likely related to the fact that the genotypes that cause acute and chronic pancreatitis only cause moderate loss of CFTR function. To date, more than 1500 CFTR mutations have been identified, most on chromosome 7. Genetic testing of patients with IARP reveals that approximately 10% to 15% of patients have CFTR mutations. As with hereditary pancreatitis, it remains unclear how the diagnosis can assist in treatment other than for family planning.

Drugs

Drug-induced acute pancreatitis is a rare entity, challenging for clinicians and often overlooked in the evaluation of patients with IARP. Although more than 120 drugs have been implicated in causing acute pancreatitis, many case reports suffer from a combina-

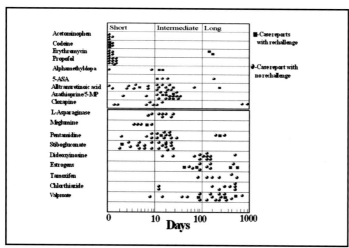

Figure 12-1. Latency of drugs with the most evidence of causing acute pancreatitis, more than 3 case reports with similar latency and those with a rechallenge. The drugs are shown with the case reports plotted as time from the initiation of drug to the onset of acute pancreatitis. Note the grouping of the drugs as immediate onset, medium, and late development of acute pancreatitis.

Table 12-3

Summary of Idiopathic Acute Recurrent Pancreatitis Additional Work-Up

- Microlithiasis—duodenal or bile aspirate
- Magnetic resonance cholangiopancreatography for pancreas divisum
- Sphincter of Oddi dysfunction—consider sphincter of Oddi manometry, endoscopic retrograde cholangiopancreatography-endoscopic sphincterotomy
- Anatomic anomalies (annular pancreas, anomalous pancreatic-biliary junction, etc)
- Genetic factors
- Drugs

---

tion of inadequate criteria for the diagnosis of acute pancreatitis, failure to rule out more common etiologies, and/or a lack of a rechallenge with the medication. Drug-induced pancreatitis rarely is accompanied by clinical or laboratory evidence of a drug reaction, such as rash, lymphadenopathy, and/or eosinophilia. Although a positive rechallenge with a drug is the best evidence available for cause and effect, it is not proof. It is clear that many patients with idiopathic pancreatitis or microlithiasis have recurrent attacks of acute pancreatitis. Therefore, stopping and restarting a drug with recurrence of pancreatitis may be a coincidence and not cause and effect. Despite the lack of a rechallenge, a drug may be strongly suspected if there is a consistent latency among the case reports between initiating the drug and the onset of acute pancreatitis. A complete review[2] is impossible here. However, the drugs with the best evidence as causing acute pancreatitis are listed in Figure 12-1.

In conclusion, IARP may be caused by a number of disorders. The most important aspect in the evaluation is not to miss the most common causes (Table 12-3), especially gallstone disease (microlithiasis). Additionally, it is important for clinicians to establish the correct diagnosis without inducing injury to patients. Further study, especially with blinded, randomized, controlled clinical trials are needed to fully address the best approach in the diagnosis and treatment of IARP. For now, a conservative approach with limited intervention is preferred.

References

1. Hogan WJ, Geenen JE. Biliary dyskenesia. *Endoscopy.* 1988;20(Suppl 1):179-183.
2. Badalov N, Baradarian R, Iswara K, Li JJ, Steinberg W, Tenner S. Drug induced acute pancreatitis: an evidence based approach. *Clinical Gastroenterology and Hepatology.* 2007;101:454-476.

Bibliography

Lehman GA. Acute recurrent pancreatitis. *Can J Gastroenterol.* 2003;17:381-383.

Levy M, Geenen J. Idiopathic acute recurrent pancreatitis. *Am J Gastroenterol.* 2001;2640-2555.

Somogyi L, Martin SP, Venkatesan T, et al. Recurrent acute pancreatitis: an algorithmic approach to identification and elimination of inciting factors. *Gastroenterology.* 2001;120:708-717.

Tenner SM, Dubner H, Steinberg W. The role of laboratory values in the diagnosis of gallstone pancreatitis: a meta-analysis. *Am J Gastroenterol.* 1994;92:323-328.

Tenner SM, Steinberg W. The lipase to amylase ratio in distinguishing alcoholic from non-alcoholic acute pancreatitis. *Am J Gastroenterol.* 1992;87:1755-1759.

How Is Hypertriglyceridemia Treated When Suspected in Causing Acute Pancreatitis?

Susan Ramdhaney, MD and Scott Tenner, MD, MPH

Hypertriglyceridemia is seen in 12% to 22% of patients presenting with acute pancreatitis. The triglycerides should only be considered the etiology when the level is over 1000 mg/dL. In these patients, the level should be rechecked 10 to 14 days after the attack of acute pancreatitis to confirm the elevation. In the setting of acute pancreatitis, the triglyceride level fluctuates for a variety of reasons. While the etiology remains unclear, proposed mechanisms in which an elevated triglyceride level causes acute pancreatitis include pancreatic acinar cell damage by free fatty acids, activation by pancreatic lipase resulting in a cascade of activated trypsinogen, and a deficiency of lipoprotein lipase and a defect in lipoprotein receptors. It is important to recognize this etiology of acute pancreatitis since initiation of proper treatment is essential for improving outcome and, more importantly, preventing recurrent attacks and the subsequent development of chronic pancreatitis.

When should we suspect hyperlipidemic pancreatitis? Three clinical syndromes have been described: (1) the poorly controlled obese diabetic with history of hypertriglyceridemia, (2) the alcoholic found to have hypertriglyceridemia or lactescent serum upon admission, and (3) the nondiabetic, nonalcoholic, nonobese patient with drug- or diet-induced hypertriglyceridemia. Hence, look for patients with a genetic predisposition such as type V hyperlipidemia (elevation of chylomicrons and very-low-density lipoprotein [VLDL]) and coexisting secondary causes of hypertriglyceridemia such as alcohol use, diabetes, hypothyroidism, uremia, nephritic syndrome, or rapid weight gain.

It is important for clinicians to obtain a good medication history since drugs that raise plasma triglycerides, such as alcohol, thiazides and loop diuretics, beta-blockers, estrogens in oral contraceptives or in post-menopausal therapy, tamoxifen, glucocorticoids, retinoids, ketogenic diets, protease inhibitors, and cimetidine, have all been implicated. Be aware of the pregnant patient since mortality from pancreatitis is even higher (20%) and you may not suspect hyperlipidemia but cholelithiasis as the etiology of acute pancreatitis. During the third trimester of pregnancy, increased synthesis of triglycerides occurs along with VLDL secretion, hyperinsulinemia, and decreased levels of apolipoprotein CII (apo-CII). Hence, with a pre-existing hyperlipidemic state, she may develop severe acute pancreatitis.

What lab values should you expect? Chylomicrons are present in plasma when triglyceride levels exceed 1000 mg/dL and are clinically significant from 1000 mg/dL to 2000 mg/dL or greater than 11.3 mmol/L. Frequently, patients have lipemic serum with normal to mildly elevated amylase and lipase and with some evidence of pancreatic inflammation on imaging studies. Hyponatremia is a frequent finding and reflects pseudohyponatremia secondary to hyperlipidemia. The lack of sensitivity and low levels of initial serum pancreatic enzymes reported may be due to the presence of an inhibitor in the blood and measuring elevated serum amylase/creatinine clearance ratios or delayed triglyceride clearance may be beneficial, but no current studies validate this.

In the acute setting, presentation of hypertriglyceridemic pancreatitis varies from mild to moderate to severe. As supportive care is initiated—nothing-by-mouth, intravenous fluids, pain management—abdominal pain may diminish and triglyceride levels may fall within the first 24 hours. However, cases of fulminant pancreatitis, pancreatic pseudocysts and abscesses, chronic pancreatitis with and without steatorrhea, and acute recurrent pancreatitis have been reported. Therefore, it is key to introduce lipid-lowering agents such as statins or fibrates early with the goal of decreasing serum triglyceride levels to less than 500 mg/dL. If the patient is diabetic, then strict glucose control with insulin is necessary. When there is no appreciable reduction in serum triglycerides, plasma exchange (replacing the patient's plasma with human albumin or fresh frozen plasma) has been used to lower excessive lipid levels, to supplement lipoprotein lipase and apolipoprotein, and to alter the cytokine balance and decrease inflammation. Studies have found that plasmaphoresis lowers plasma lipids by two-thirds in about 2 hours (triglycerides by 66%, cholesterol by 62%) and clears them to less than 1000 mg/dL with improvement of abdominal pain. However, experience with plasmaphoresis is limited in hyperlipidemic pancreatitis patients even though it is an established treatment for familial hypercholesterolemia. Some studies also advocate the use of heparin and insulin to stimulate lipoprotein lipase and chylomicron degradation, thereby decreasing triglyceride levels with resolution of pancreatitis. The data, however, are limited.

How should we manage these patients once they are discharged? Focus on preventing recurrent attacks of acute pancreatitis with chronic lipid-lowering medications and diet modification. Maintenance therapy with gemfibrozil 600 mg bid, clofibrate 1 g bid, nicotinic acid 500 mg qd increased to 3 to 6 g qd as well as omega-3 fatty acids with 5% to 15% total calories fish oil should be employed. Diet modification with substitution of saturated fat with polyunsaturated fat and starch and fiber for sucrose-containing foods should be initiated. Strict glycemic control should be maintained in diabetic patients and weight loss with aerobic exercise encouraged. Pancreatic serine proteinases such as gabexate mesylate which decreases pancreatic stimulation through feedback inhibition and loxiglumide, a cholecystokinin receptor antagonist, have been suggested for use until triglyceride levels fall to less than 500 mg. However, no ultrasound study supports this practice. Some suggest that plasmaphoresis performed every 4 weeks decreases the incidence of pancreatitis but this too is controversial.

In summary, proper management of hypertriglyceridemic pancreatitis lies in the ability to recognize the disease (resist the temptation to label as idiopathic pancreatitis) and to lower serum triglycerides early in its course. Start lipid-lowering medications as an inpatient and continue prevention of hyperchylomicronemia as an outpatient. Encourage dietary restriction of triglycerides, weight loss, diabetic control, exercise, and the avoidance of alcohol and drugs known to increase serum triglycerides. With this in mind, we can work toward decreasing the incidence of hypertriglyceridemic pancreatitis and improving the outcome.

Bibliography

Fortson MR, Freedman SN, Webster PD III. Clinical assessment of hyperlipidemic pancreatitis. *Am J Gastroenterol.* 1995;90(12):2134-2139.

Lennertz A, Parhofer KG, Samtleben W, Bosch T. Therapeutic plasma exchange in patients with chylomicronemia syndrome, complicated by acute pancreatitis. *Therap Apher.* 1999;3:227-233.

Piolot A, Jacotot B, et al. Prevention of recurrent acute pancreatitis in patients with severe hypertriglyceridemia: value of regular plasmaphoresis. *Pancreas.* 1996;13(1):96-99.

Toskes PP. Hyperlipidemic pancreatitis. *Gastroenterol Clin North Am.* 1990;19:783-791.

My Patient With Crohn's Disease Developed Pancreatitis on Imuran. Can He Take 6-MP?

Nison Badalov, MD and Scott Tenner, MD, MPH

Drug-induced acute pancreatitis is a rare entity that often is challenging for clinicians. Although more than 120 drugs have been implicated in causing acute pancreatitis, many case reports suffer from a combination of inadequate criteria for the diagnosis of acute pancreatitis, failure to rule out more common causes, and/or a lack of a rechallenge with the medication. Drug-induced pancreatitis rarely is accompanied by clinical or laboratory evidence of a drug reaction, such as rash, lymphadenopathy, and/or eosinophilia. Although a positive rechallenge with a drug is the best evidence available for cause and effect, it is not proof. It is clear that many patients with idiopathic pancreatitis or microlithiasis have recurrent attacks of acute pancreatitis. Therefore, stopping and restarting a drug with recurrence of pancreatitis may be a coincidence and not cause and effect. Despite the lack of a rechallenge, a drug may be strongly suspected if there is a consistent latency among the case reports between initiating the drug and the onset of acute pancreatitis.

Azathioprine and its metabolite, 6-mercaptopurine (6-MP), have strong evidence implicating them as agents that cause acute pancreatitis (Table 14-1). In the National Cooperative Crohn's Disease Study, almost 6% of 116 patients treated with azathioprine developed acute pancreatitis. During a 15-year period, from 1969 to 1985, Haber et al[1] treated 400 patients with inflammatory bowel with 6-MP. Thirteen (3.25%) developed acute pancreatitis thought to be related to the medication. There are 20 case reports of acute pancreatitis resulting from therapy with azathioprine and 6-MP. Four definite cases (confirmed by computed tomography and ultrasound) have had positive rechallenge, 3 with azathioprine and 1 with 6-MP. All 4 cases of acute pancreatitis occurred 2 to 4 weeks after initiating 50 to 100 mg/dL of the drug, and recurrence of pancreatitis occurred within 2 days of rechallenge. Although these 4 cases had mild disease, there are reports of severe acute pancreatitis in patients taking these antimetabolites. Renning,[2] Hamed,[3] Kolk,[4] and their

Table 14-1

Summary of Case Reports of Azathioprine, 6-Mercaptopurine Causing Acute Pancreatitis With Rechallenge

Drug	Case(s)	Dosage(s)	Latency	Repeat Latency	Definite/ Probable	Outcome
Azathioprine	3	50 mg/d	27 days	2 days	Definite	Mild
		100 mg/d	20 days	1 day	Definite	Mild
6-Mercaptopurine	1	100 mg/d	17 days	Rapid	Definite	Mild

colleagues report 5 patients whose pancreatitis was severe, resulting in infection, hemorrhage, pseudocyst, and death.

There are several potential pathogenetic mechanisms of drug-induced pancreatitis. The most common is a hypersensitivity reaction. This tends to occur 4 to 8 weeks after starting the drug and is not a dose-related phenomenon. Upon rechallenge with the drug, pancreatitis re-occurs within hours to days. Examples of drugs that operate through this mechanism are 6-MP/azathioprine, aminosalicylates, metronidazole, and tetracycline. The second mechanism is the presumed accumulation of a toxic metabolite that may cause pancreatitis. Typically, drugs like these cause pancreatitis after several months of usage. Examples of drugs in this category are valproic acid and didanosine. Drugs that induce hypertriglyceridemia (thiazides, isotretinoin, tamoxifen, etc) are also in this category. Finally, very few drugs may have intrinsic toxicity wherein an overdose can cause pancreatitis (erythromycin, acetaminophen). There is no documentation that drugs can cause pancreatitis after years of usage.

In summary, drug-induced pancreatitis due to 6-MP and azathioprine tends to be mild and self-limited, occurring between 2 and 4 weeks after initiation with almost an immediate repeat latency if rechallenged. There are no cases in which a patient had a bout of acute pancreatitis to either 6-MP or azathioprine and then were challenged with the other medication. However, as 6-MP is the metabolite of azathioprine and all subsequent metabolites that cause other side effects reported (such as bone marrow suppression) are the same, it would be likely that the biologic mechanisms that induce acute pancreatitis are the same and thus both medications should be avoided if the attack of acute pancreatitis is truly believed to be related to either 6-MP or azathioprine.

References

1. Haber CJ, Meltzer SJ, Present DH, Korelitz BI. Nature and course of pancreatitis caused by 6-mercoptopurine in the treatment of inflammatory bowel disease. *Gastroenterology.* 1986;91:982-986.
2. Renning JA, Warden GD, Stevens LE, Reemstsma K. Pancreatitis after renal transplantation. *Am J Med.* 1972;123:293-296.
3. Hamed I, Linderman RD, Czerwinski AW. Acute pancreatitis following corticosteroid and azathioprine therapy. *Am J Med Sci.* 1978;276:211-219.
4. Kolk A, Horneff G, Wilgenbus KK, Wahn V, Gerharz CD. Acute lethal necrotizing pancreatitis in childhood systemic lupus erythematosus—possible toxicity of immunosuppressive therapy. *Clin Exp Rheumatol.* 1995;13(3):399-403.

Bibliography

Badalov N, Baradarian R, Iswara K, Li JJ, Steinberg W, Tenner S. Drug induced acute pancreatits: an evidence based approach. *Clinical Gastroenterology and Hepatology.* 2007;101:454-476.

Present DH, Korelitz BI, Wisch N, Glass JL, Sachar DB, Pasternack BS. Treatment of Crohn's desease with 6-mercaptopurine. *N Engl J Med.* 1980;302:981-987.

MY PATIENT WITH ACUTE PANCREATITIS HAS A COMPUTED TOMOGRAPHY SCAN WITH THROMBOSIS OF THE SPLENIC VEIN. IS IT SAFE TO ANTICOAGULATE HIM?

Susan Ramdhaney, MD and Alphonso Brown, MD, MS Clin Epi

Isolated thrombosis of the splenic vein occurs as a result of left-sided portal hypertension and due to complications from acute and chronic pancreatitis, pancreatic cancer, adenopathy from metastatic cancer, or from iatrogenic causes such as splenectomy, partial gastrectomy, and distal splenorenal shunt. As a complication of chronic pancreatitis, which occurs in 3% to 5% of cases, it should be suspected in patients with a history of pancreatitis and gastrointestinal blood loss; a patient with splenomegaly in the absence of portal hypertension, cirrhosis, or hematologic disease; and in the setting of isolated gastric varices.

Splenic vein thrombosis is often detected after a severe bout of acute pancreatitis during the evaluation of foci of pancreatic necrosis (Figure 15-1). Diagnostic tests of splenic vein thrombosis include celiac angiography which has replaced splenoportography as the definitive diagnostic tool for splenic vein thrombosis and is indicated prior to operation for suspected portal hypertension or for complications of pancreatitis. However, endoscopic ultrasonography (EUS) has emerged as a fairly sensitive and noninvasive diagnostic tool. EUS can help determine the presence of perigastric varices which are the anatomical problems that result in upper gastrointestinal bleeding (Figure 15-2).

Rarely, thrombosis of the splenic vein may be discovered many years after the episode of pancreatitis where the affected individual presents with an acute upper gastrointestinal bleed and associated gastric varices which develop as a secondary compensatory

Figure 15-1. Computed tomography of the abdomen in a patient with splenic vein thrombosis complicating chronic panceatitis. No varices noted.

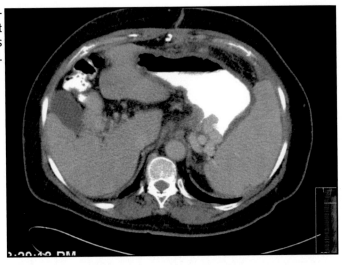

Figure 15-2. In the same patient, endoscopic ultrasound showing gastric varices which pose a great risk to spontaneous gastrointestinal bleeding.

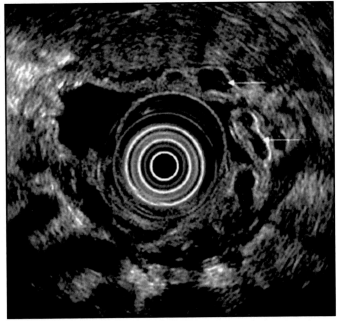

mechanism due to the increased sinestrial pressure associated with the thrombosed splenic vein. Mortality due to an acute variceal bleed in the setting of a splenic vein thrombosis can be quite high. Another worrisome complication of splenic vein thrombosis is the development of a ruptured spleen. In rare cases, splenic rupture can occur suddenly, resulting in a life-threatening intraperitoneal bleed. Due to the potentially fatal complications associated with splenic vein thrombosis, there has been much interest in the natural history of individuals who develop splenic vein thrombosis after an attack of acute pancreatitis.

One of the largest studies to date, performed by Heider et al,[1] examined the natural history of splenic vein thrombosis in a cohort of 53 patients. They eventually found that lifetime risk of variceal bleeding from isolated splenic varices varied from 5% to 18%. The potentially lethal nature of variceal bleeding has led to the recommendation to prevent the occurrence of long-term bleeding complications by prophylactic splenectomy. Though a relatively safe procedure, patients who undergo splenectomy are at an increased long-term risk of malignancy and complications associated with infection. Splenic artery embolization is being investigated in patients with high operative risk and diffuse metastatic disease, however, it may be associated with splenic vein abscess.

Acute splenic vein thrombosis most often is clinically silent and resolves spontaneously with recanalization. The risk of recurrence is not well studied. For thrombosis that does not resolve spontaneously, we need to weigh the risks of bleeding from possible gastric variceal formation vs the benefit of possible recanalization for patients who cannot undergo surgery and need alternative therapy.

Anticoagulation is an attractive alternative to surgery but at present, it remains unclear whether long-term anticoagulation for splenic vein thrombosis provides improved outcomes over splenectomy. Evidence-based medicine supports the use of anticoagulation for portal vein thrombosis. There is not enough evidence to support or reject anticoagulation for splenic vein thrombosis. Condat et al[2] evaluated 33 patients with acute portal vein thrombosis presenting with no evidence of portal hypertension and no portal collaterals on imaging. Patients received heparin/Coumadin (Bristol-Myers Squibb, New York, NY) and had follow-up imaging. Most patients had recanalization but 2 patients who received no anticoagulation showed no recanalization. Based on this study, it appears that individuals with thrombosed portal veins should be treated with anticoagulants. We assume that patients with splenic vein thrombosis will also benefit. However, there are no guidelines as to the dose or length of treatment needed for splenic vein thrombosis. Treatment should be individualized for each patient.

Based on these data, it would appear that anticoagulation is a safe option for patients with chronic splenic vein thrombosis due to pancreatitis who are at increased risk of complications from the sequelae of chronic isolated splenic vein thrombosis. However, it remains unclear whether this will be more effective than a strategy of observation or splenectomy.

References

1. Heider R, Behrns KE. Pancreatic pseudocysts complicated by splenic parenchymal involvement: results of operative and percutaneous management. *Pancreas.* 2001;23(1):20-25.
2. Condat B, Pessione F, Helene DM, et al. Recent portal or mesenteric thrombosis: increased recognition and frequent recanalization on anticoagulant therapy. *Hepatology.* 2000;32:466-470.

Bibliography

Kakizaki S, Hamada T, Yoshinaga T, et al. Alcoholic chronic pancreatitis with simultaneous multiple severe complications—extrahepatic portal obliteration, obstructive jaundice and duodenal stricture. *Hepatogastroenterology.* 2005;52(64):1274-1277.

Simpson WG, Schwartz RW, Strodel WE. Splenic vein thrombosis. *South Med J.* 1990;83(4):417-421.

Weber SM, Rikkers LF. Splenic vein thrombosis and gastrointestinal bleeding in chronic pancreatitis. *World J Surg.* 2003;27(11):1271-1274.

SECTION II

CHRONIC PANCREATITIS

HOW IS THE DIAGNOSIS OF CHRONIC PANCREATITIS ESTABLISHED?

Jonathan Ari Erber, MD and Frank G. Gress, MD

Chronic pancreatitis is a syndrome of progressive destructive inflammatory changes in the pancreas that results in permanent structural damage, which leads to impairment of exocrine and endocrine function.[1] Histologic changes include irregular fibrosis, acinar cell loss, islet cell loss, and inflammatory cell infiltrates. The gold standard for the diagnosis of chronic pancreatitis is tissue, however, this is invasive and rarely performed. Therefore, the diagnosis of chronic pancreatitis is based upon a combination of clinical, radiographic, and functional findings.

The hallmark manifestations of chronic pancreatitis are abdominal pain and exocrine insufficiency. Abdominal pain is the most common presenting complaint, seen in 50% to 90% of patients. The pain is typically epigastric, radiates to the back, is worse after meals, and may be relieved by sitting upright or leaning forward (pancreatic position). Early in the course, the pain may be intermittent and occur in discrete attacks, but as the disease progresses, the pain becomes more continuous. Severe pain may decrease the appetite and limit food consumption, which contributes to weight loss and malnutrition.

Exocrine insufficiency is generally not seen until at least 90% of the pancreas has been destroyed, first with fat and later protein and carbohydrate maldigestion with steatorrhea. Patients may note bulky, foul-smelling stools or even the passage of frank oily droplets. Diabetes occurs late in the course of chronic pancreatitis. The diabetes is often brittle with frequent episodes of hypoglycemia, due to the destruction of both the beta cells as well as the glucagon-producing alpha cells.

We generally obtain routine labs including liver function tests, which are often normal. Amylase and lipase may be normal and if elevated, typically only minimally so. Serum trypsinogen, which is very low (<20 ng/mL) in chronic pancreatitis is specific but not sensitive. This test is commercially available and inexpensive. We do not routinely obtain this as a result of the poor sensitivity.

Table 16-1

Imaging Tests Used in the Diagnosis of Chronic Pancreatitis

Modality	Findings	Sensitivity	Specificity
KUB	Diffuse pancreatic calcification	30%	100%
US	Dilatation of the pancreatic duct	50% to 80%	80% to 90%
	Presence of pancreatic ductal stones		
	Gland atrophy or enlargement		
	Irregular gland margins		
	Pseudocysts		
	Changes in the parenchymal echotexture		
CT	Calcifications within the pancreatic ducts or parenchyma	75% to 90%	85%
	Dilated main pancreatic ducts		
	Parenchymal atrophy		
MRCP		**	**
ERCP		70% to 90%	80% to 100%
EUS		73%	81%

CT=computed tomography, ERCP=endoscopic retrograde cholangiopancreatography, EUS=endoscopic ultrasound, KUB=kidneys, ureters, and bladder, MRCP=magnetic resonance cholangiopancreatography, US=ultrasound.

In patients with diarrhea, we test the stool for qualitative fecal fat, with Sudan staining. Six globules per high power field is considered positive. It tests positive only in patients with significant steatorrhea. Fecal fat excretion over a 72-hour period may also be measured, but is often difficult to collect. The patient must follow a diet containing 100 g/day fat for at least 3 days before the test. Less than 7 g of fat (7%) is considered normal. Initial studies suggested that fecal elastase could detect mild to moderate chronic pancreatitis (without steatorrhea); however, more recent studies have shown it to be accurate only in advanced chronic pancreatitis.

Direct tests of pancreatic secretion can also be performed, but are generally only available in specialized centers. These tests are invasive, time consuming, and expensive. These tests are most useful in patients with presumed chronic pancreatitis in whom easily identifiable structural and functional abnormalities have not been demonstrated.

Functional testing for abnormalities of the pancreas, while useful in the diagnostic work-up for chronic pancreatitis, do not differentiate between pancreatic insufficiency caused by chronic pancreatitis or present without chronic pancreatitis. Therefore, imaging tests are also needed to detect the various morphologic changes associated with chronic pancreatitis and further support its diagnosis. A number of radiologic studies have been used to further define the diagnosis (Table 16-1).

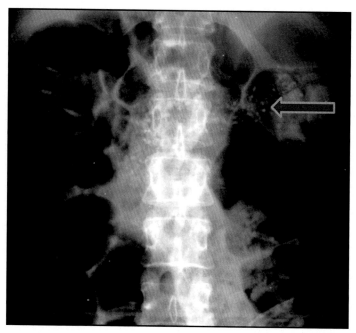

Figure 16-1. Diffuse pancreatic calcification.

Flat Plate of Abdomen

Diffuse pancreatic calcification seen on kidneys, ureters, and bladder (KUB) is almost 100% specific but not sensitive, only seen in up to 30% of patients. Although typically a KUB is not an ordered diagnostic test for the disease, the finding of diffuse calcifications is so specific for the disease (Figure 16-1).

Abdominal Ultrasound

Findings suggestive of chronic pancreatitis include dilatation of the pancreatic duct, presence of pancreatic ductal stones, gland atrophy or enlargement, irregular gland margins, pseudocysts, and changes in the parenchymal echotexture.[2] Sensitivity ranges from 50% to 80% with a specificity of 80% to 90%. The limitation is that the pancreas cannot always be adequately visualized in some due to overlying bowel gas or body habitus.

Computed Tomography of the Abdomen

This procedure is noninvasive, widely available, and has a very good sensitivity for diagnosing moderate to severe chronic pancreatitis, ranging from 75% to 90%, with a specificity of 85% or more.[2] Findings suggestive of chronic pancreatitis include calcifications within the pancreatic ducts or parenchyma and/or dilated main pancreatic ducts combined with parenchymal atrophy (Figure 16-2). Optimal evaluation of the pancreas is with helical CT using thin, 5-mm slices of the pancreas (pancreatic protocol), which is available in most tertiary referral centers. Water is used as an oral contrast agent; the

Figure 16-2. Calcification within the pancreatic duct and parenchyma, dilated pancreatic duct, and parenchymal trophy.

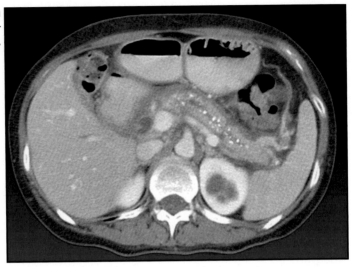

initial scan should be without intravenous contrast in order to detect pancreatic calcifications; about 150 mL of intravenous contrast is then rapidly infused, with sections obtained 35 to 40 seconds later (pancreatic phase) and 60 to 70 seconds later (liver/portal venous phase). CT will also detect complications including pseudocysts, pseudoaneurysm, and biliary obstruction. The presence of pancreatic head enlargement may suggest cancer or an inflammatory mass.

Magnetic Resonance Imaging and Magnetic Resonance Cholangiopancreatography of the Abdomen

The role of MRI of the abdomen and MRCP in the diagnosis of chronic pancreatitis is evolving. Presently, MRI of the abdomen is not routinely performed unless there is a contraindication to the use of intravenous contrast with CT. Its advantages are that it is noninvasive, avoids ionizing radiation and intravenous contrast administration, and does not routinely require sedation. MRCP results correlate fairly well with endoscopic retrograde cholangiopancreatography (ERCP), in the range of 70% to 80% of cases (Figure 16-3). MRCP may be useful in patients with gastric outlet obstruction, duodenal stenosis, altered surgical anatomy, such as an Roux-en-Y, or Billroth II anatomy.

Endoscopic Retrograde Cholangiopancreatography

If clinical suspicion remains high, and noninvasive imaging fails to support the diagnosis of chronic pancreatitis, we perform ERCP or endoscopic ultrasound (EUS). ERCP is widely available and has the advantage that it allows for therapeutic interventions (ie, pancreatic duct stenting or stone extraction). In the absence of a tissue diagnosis, ERCP

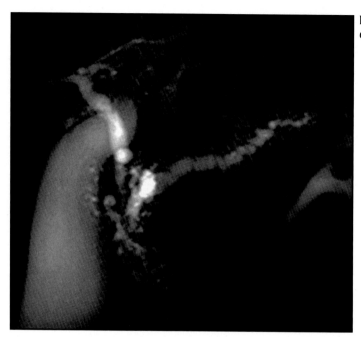

Figure 16-3. Dilated and tortuous pancreatic duct.

Table 16-2

Cambridge Classification

Grade	Main Pancreatic Duct	Side Branches
Normal	Normal	Normal
Equivocal	Normal	<3 Abnormal
Mild	Normal	≥3 Abnormal
Moderate	Abnormal	≥3 Abnormal

Severe	Abnormal with at least 1 of the following:
	    Large cavity (>10 mm)
	    Obstruction
	    Filling defects
	    Severe dilatation or irregularity
		≥3 Abnormal

is considered the gold standard with a sensitivity of 70% to 90% and specificity of 80% to 100%. In mild or early disease, findings include dilatation and irregularity of the smaller ducts and branches of the pancreatic duct. In moderate disease, these changes are also found in the main pancreatic duct. With increasing severity, tortuosity, stricture, calcification, and cysts are also seen. The degree of chronic pancreatitis can be determined by the number of abnormalities found at ERCP (Cambridge classification [Table 16-2]).[2] ERCP is relatively invasive, with a complication rate of around 7% to 10%.[3] It requires a high level of operator experience, with substantial inter- and intra-observer variability in interpretation of mild to moderate disease.

Figure 16-4. Hyperechoic foci and strands, lobularity, and main duct dilatation.

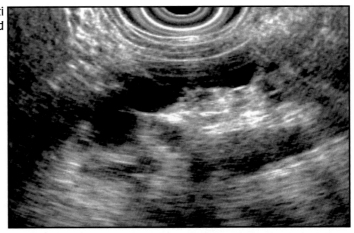

Table 16-3
Diagnosis of Chronic Pancreatitis on Endoscopic Ultrasound

Parenchymal abnormalities	Hyperechoic foci
	Hyperechoic strands
	Lobular contour
	Cysts
Ductal abnormalities	Main duct dilatation
	Irregularity
	Hyperechoic margins
	Dilated side branches
	Stones

Endoscopic Ultrasound

The role of EUS is evolving but is taking on an increasingly more important role in the diagnosis and management of chronic pancreatitis (Figure 16-4 and Table 16-3). High-resolution images of the parenchyma and pancreatic duct can be obtained using a high frequency radial or linear EUS probe (ranges between 5 and 20 MHz) fixed on the tip of an endoscope and placed in close approximation to the pancreas. The EUS instrument is inserted through the esophagus into the stomach and duodenum and manipulated to obtain high-quality images of the head/uncinate process, body, and tail of the pancreas. EUS can also be used to obtain tissue using EUS-guided fine needle aspiration technique for cytology or a true cut core biopsy needle for histology. The diagnosis is based upon the presence of abnormalities in the pancreatic duct and parenchyma similar to abdominal ultrasound. EUS sensitivity approaches 73% and specificity 81% depending on the diagnostic criteria used. EUS and ERCP agree in about 80% of patients.[4,5] The disadvantages to this modality are that it is not widely available and highly operator dependent.

In summary, the diagnosis of chronic pancreatitis is based upon a combination of clinical, radiographic, and functional findings. Although secretin stimulation pancreatic function testing is sensitive and specific, the limited availability of this modality forces clinicians to rely on structural testing. Although KUB and CT are specific, they are not sensitive. MRI with MRCP is sensitive and specific and noninvasive. MRI should be performed initially, with EUS and ERCP reserved for those patients with an equivocal diagnosis.

References

1. Etemad B, Whitcomb DC. Chronic pancreatitis: diagnosis, classification, and new genetic developments. *Gastroenterology.* 2001;120:682-688.
2. Axon AT, Classen M, Cotton PB, et al. Pancreatography in chronic pancreatitis: international definitions. *Gut.* 2004;25:1107-1121.
3. Freeman ML, DiSario JA, Nelson DB, et al. Risk factors for post-ERCP pancreatitis: a prospective, multicenter study. *Gastrointest Endosc.* 2001;54:425-434.
4. Sahai AV, Zimmerman M, Aabakken L, et al. Prospective assessment of the ability of endoscopic ultrasound to diagnose, exclude, or establish the severity of chronic pancreatitis found by endoscopic retrograde cholangiopancreatography. *Gastrointest Endosc.* 1998;48:18-25.
5. Wallace MB, Hawes RH, Durkalski V, et al. The reliability of EUS for the diagnosis of chronic pancreatitis: interobserver agreement among experienced endosonographers. *Gastrointest Endosc.* 2001;53:294-299.

WHAT IS THE BEST METHOD OF TREATING PAIN IN PATIENTS WITH CHRONIC PANCREATITIS?

Kumaravel Perumalsamy, MD and Scott Tenner, MD, MPH

It has been estimated that the pain complicating chronic pancreatitis results in 5 billion dollars a year in excess direct health care costs and an additional 50 billion dollars in loss of productivity. Painful chronic pancreatitis is poorly understood and its management is controversial.[1] Our lack of knowledge about what causes pain in pancreatitis has been a serious obstacle to improvement of the care of these patients. Unfortunately, most approaches are empirical, often based on purely anatomical issues, and often highly invasive and at best of marginal value. Despite a wide variety of approaches—innocuous (enzyme therapy), minimally invasive (endoscopic decompression, nerve blocks) and highly aggressive (surgical decompression, pancreatectomy)—no consensus has emerged and no form of treatment can be considered satisfactory at the present time.

The pain in chronic pancreatitis can vary highly from patient to patient as well as over time in the same patient. The mechanism of pain in chronic pancreatitis is incompletely understood and perhaps multifactorial, including inflammation, duct obstruction, high pancreatic tissue pressure (compartment syndrome), fibrotic encasement of sensory nerves, and a neuropathy characterized by both increased numbers and sizes of intra-pancreatic sensory nerves and by inflammatory injury to the nerve sheaths allowing exposure of the neural elements to toxic substances. Several factors may contribute to this variability, including etiology, natural history of the pancreatitis, and the presence or the absence of associated complications (eg, pseudocysts, biliary obstruction). According to Cahen et al,[2] pain will develop in approximately 75% of patients with alcoholic chronic pancreatitis, 50% of patients with late-onset idiopathic chronic pancreatitis, and 100% of patients with early-onset idiopathic chronic pancreatitis. The view that chronic pain will subside in a substantial number of patients with or without organ failure as the disease progress to the point of organ failure (burnout) has been widely accepted, but that process

Table 17-1

Current Approaches to the Management of Pain in Chronic Pancreatitis

1. General measures
   a. Cessation of alcohol intake
   b. Analgesics
2. Reduction of intrapancreatic pressure
   a. Suppression of secretion
      i. Enzymes
      ii. Octreotide
   b. Decompression techniques
      i. Endoscopic dilatation and stenting
      ii. Stone removal (endoscopic or extracorporeal shock wave lithotripsy)
   c. Surgical drainage (Peustow)
3. Organ resection
4. Neural interruption
   a. Percutaneous or endoscopic (EUS) nerve blocks
   b. Surgical (thorascopic) splanchnic nerve resection

may take an unpredictable number of years or may never occur. A decision to withhold surgical or other invasive therapies in the hope of eventual burnout is probably not warranted. One series reported spontaneous cessation of pain in only about 25% of patients over an 8-year period.[3]

The management of pain in chronic pancreatitis requires skill and patience, as well as a clear and realistic understanding of the goals of the treatment and a firm "patient-physician" relationship. The care should involve a multidisciplinary team including pain management services, mental health professionals, anesthesiologists, and social and rehabilitation workers. However, the gastroenterologist remains central in this process and familiarity with the principles and practice of chronic narcotic prescriptions is essential. In general, the approaches of treatment are aimed a decreasing pancreatic ductal pressure. The current approaches to the treatment of pain in chronic pancreatitis are conceptually summarized in Table 17-1 and will be discussed in detail.

Medical Treatment

Medical treatment of pancreatic endocrine and exocrine function has been largely successful through the control of diabetes with insulin and malabsorption with pancreatic enzyme supplementation. However, the medical treatment of pain has led to poor results. Narcotics are useful for brief episodes of pain, however, long-term use leads to tachyphylaxis and resistance requiring escalating doses and in some cases addiction.

Pancreatic enzymes are of little value in the management of pain. The rationale behind enzyme treatment is that activated proteinases in the duodenal lumen cleave the peptide that causes release of cholecystokinin (CCK) and hence suppress further pancreatic secretion, diminishing intraductal pressure. Only 1 of 6 of randomized controlled trials showed a statistically significant benefit and only 52% of the pooled patient population expressing a preference for enzyme over placebo.[4] In general, pancreatic enzymes only provide a placebo effect in the treatment of pain. Although there has been some study regarding the use of octreotide, the response to octreotide in this setting has similarly been disappointing.

Endoscopic Approaches

Endoscopic approaches are used in many patients as an alternative to surgery for the treatment of pseudocysts, stone removal, stricture dilatation/stenting, or pancreatic sphincter hypertension. The concept is based on the importance of decompression of the pancreatic duct to prevent theoretical pancreatic ductal hypertension produced by the obstruction. The idea is that the pain is caused by the blockage of the pancreatic duct and thus removing the obstruction will relieve the pain. Stricture dilatation and stenting have been reported to vary widely in efficacy, with persistent pain relief ranging from as low as 11% to nearly 90%[2]; this variation in part is explained by the divergent nature of the trials and methodology as well as the underlying pathology and techniques used. Endoscopic stone removal combined with extracorporeal shock wave lithotripsy (ESWL) has clearly been shown to be effective in relieving pain in a subset of patients with chronic calcific pancreatitis. Following ESWL and stone clearance, pain relief varies from approximately 50% to 80% (Figure 17-1). In addition, endoscopic drainage of pseudocysts into the stomach and duodenum is now widely practiced and is often effective in relieving pain in patients with this complication.[5]

Sensory pancreatic nerves pass through the celiac ganglion. After noting some success with computed tomography (CT)-guided blocks, a real time endoscopic approach with endoscopic ultrasound (EUS) has been developed. This technique involves injection of neurolytic chemicals such as alcohol, steroids, or phenol. Celiac plexus block typically consists of the use of a local anesthetic such as bupivacaine, usually along with a steroid. These agents are short acting with effects that range from a few days to months at most. True neurolytic injections use toxic chemicals such as absolute alcohol or phenol that cause permanent damage to the nerves. However, permanence is seldom if ever achieved in practice and most investigators avoid the use of alcohol for fear of potential neurological consequences such as paraplegia.

EUS-guided celiac plexus block was more effective, as attested by the proportion of patients reporting short-term relief (50% vs 25%) and also less expensive ($1100 vs $1400) than CT-guided celiac plexus block.[6] However, the percutaneous method may be the preferred method for the occasional patient who is at high risk for conscious sedation or general anesthesia. In general, the response rate for EUS-guided celiac plexus block was poorer in younger patients (<45 years), and those with a history of prior pancreatic surgery for chronic pancreatitis were least likely to benefit.

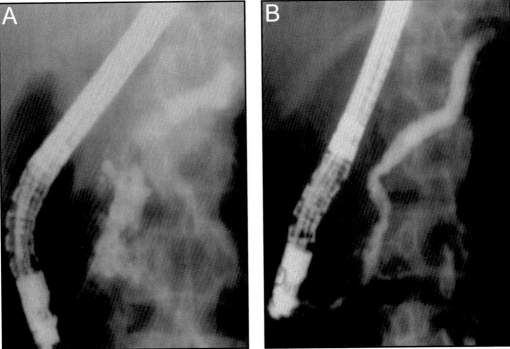

Figure 17-1. Results and endsocopic approach of painful chronic pancreatitis. Endoscopic retrograde cholangiopancreatography before (A) and after treatment (B) with extracorporeal shock wave lithotripsy. Note excellent results opening duct. Patient remains pain free following therapy.

Surgical Approaches

Surgical approaches are clearly effective in carefully selected patients in whom dilated ducts or obvious inflammatory disease exist. The first widely used surgical approach for painful pancreatitis was the lateral pancreatojejunostomy. Although first described by Puestow and Gillesby[7] and modified by Partington and Rochelle,[8] this is a decompression procedure. The ideal patient has a dilated dorsal duct (Santorini) which cannot be stented from the minor or major papilla. By opening the pancreas (a fillet procedure) and relieving putative high intrapancreatic pressures as is implied by the presence of significant dilated main pancreatic duct (>6 to 7 mm), pain relief is expected. Short-term results with this procedure are impressive; pain relief is achieved in 80% of cases with very low morbidity and mortality (0% to 5%). However, these results are not sustained over time: as early as 2 years after surgery, pain relief persists in only 60% of patients with perhaps a further decline in the long term. These procedures are probably best done by experts in major referral centers. A recent study by Cahen and colleagues[2] suggested that this approach was superior to endoscopic stenting/stone removal. However, Elta,[5] in an eloquent editorial, discusses the importance of considering less invasive endoscopic therapy initially and the importance of patient selection.

Patients without dilated ducts (small duct disease) do not have the same decompressive options, either endoscopically or surgically. Surgical options are aimed at removing the inflammatory mass and include the Whipple procedure or pylorus-preserving pancreaticoduodenectomy, distal pancreatectomy, or total pancreatectomy. Resection of the pancreatic head by either a conventional or pylorus-preserving pancreaticoduodenectomy will provide pain relief in up to 85% of patients, even if the disease extends into the distal pancreas. Again, however, long-term results may not be sustained and fall to 50% to 70%. Duodenum-preserving resection of the pancreatic head in patients with inflammatory masses in the head of the pancreas with short-term pain relief were reported in 70% to 90% of cases. Distal pancreatectomy alone has poor results unless the disease is largely confined to the body and tail of the gland. While theoretically able to provide complete relief, total pancreatectomy is not recommended because not only do a significant number of patients continue to have pain, but the metabolic consequences can be very severe. Although autotransplantation of islet or pancreatic tissue is being performed in combination with this procedure in some centers, low success rates and technical challenges remain formidable obstacles. Surgery may be considered superior to endotherapy for long-term pain reduction in patients with painful obstructive chronic pancreatitis.

Thoracoscopic splanchnectomy is a recent surgical approach to neural interruption. Initial studies are promising but further study is needed. The risks of this procedure include atelectasis, intercostal neuralgias, pneumothorax, chlyothorax, bleeding, postural hypotension, and pneumonia. It is not practiced outside major medical centers.

In summary, painful chronic pancreatitis remains a major clinical challenge. Management of these patients is difficult. All current available measures have significant shortcomings. Although long-term use of narcotics is not warranted due to tachyphylaxis and the need for dose escalation, short-term use can be beneficial. Pancreatic enzymes have no role for the treatment of pain. Endoscopic or surgical decompression of a stricture, obstructed and dilated pancreatic duct, and/or pseudocyst is effective in a majority of patients. In the absence of an obvious lesion to decompress, EUS with celiac axis block can be effective in select patients. Careful patient evaluation, selection of intervention based on imaging and expertise, and a clear discussion of risks and benefits to any intervention are paramount in managing pain in patients with chronic pancreatitis.

References

1. Dimagno EP. Toward understanding (and management) of painful chronic pancreatitis. *Gastroenterology.* 1999;116:1252-1257.
2. Cahen DL, Gouma DJ, Nio Y, et al. Endoscopic versus surgical drainage of the pancreatic duct in chronic pancreatitis. *N Engl J Med.* 2007;356:676-684.
3. Lankisch PG, Seidensticker F, Lohr-Happe A, Otto J, Creutzfeldt W. The course of pain is the same in alcohol and nonalcohol-induced chronic pancreatitis. *Pancreas.* 1995;10:338-341.
4. Brown A, Hughes M, Tenner S, Banks PA. Does pancreatic enzyme supplementation reduce pain in patients with chronic pancreatitis: a meta-analysis. *Am J Gastroenterol.* 1997;92:2032-2035.
5. Elta G. Is there a role for the endoscopic treatment of pain from chronic pancreatitis? *N Engl J Med.* 2007;27:2103-2104.
6. Gress F, Schmitt C, Sherman S, Ikenberry S, Lehman G. A prospective randomized comparison of EUS and CT guided celiac plexus block for managing chronic pancreatitis pain. *Am J Gastroenterol.* 1999;94:900-905.
7. Puestow CB, Gillesby WJ. Retrograde surgical drainage of pancreas for chronic pancreatitis. *Arch Surg.* 1958;76:898-906.
8. Partington PF, Rochelle REL. Modified Puestow procedure for retrograde drainage of the pancreatic duct. *Ann Surg.* 1960;152:1037-1043.

Is There a Role of Pancreatic Enzymes to Treat Pain in Patients With Chronic Pancreatitis?

Sagar Garud, MD, MS and Alphonso Brown, MD, MS Clin Epi

Chronic pancreatitis is associated with severe abdominal pain with episodic flares. It ranges from occasional abdominal pain associated with meals to severe incapacitating pain. The goals of enzyme therapy include pain relief and correcting the exocrine insufficiency. Pain management should be individualized for every patient and should be carried out in a stepwise manner. It is important to make sure that the pain is not due to complications of chronic pancreatitis like pseudocyst, biliary stricture, or pancreatic carcinoma. Cessation of alcohol intake is important; however, it may not always lead to pain relief.

The mechanism for pain in chronic pancreatitis is as follows. Cholecystokinin (CCK) stimulates secretion from exocrine pancreas. Pancreatic enzyme trypsin degrades CCK. In chronic pancreatitis, there is deficiency of trypsin and hence CCK is not degraded. The stimulation of pancreas by CCK leads to pain. This theory forms the basis for the use of pancreatic enzymes for pain relief in chronic pancreatitis.

There have been 6 randomized controlled trials studying the use of pancreatic enzymes in chronic pancreatitis for pain relief (Table 18-1). Two studies showed that pancreatic enzymes decrease pain in the majority of patients with chronic pancreatitis while 4 showed that they do not. A meta-analysis of these 6 trials showed that pancreatic enzymes are not effective in pain relief in chronic pancreatitis. However, this meta-analysis was limited by factors such as differences in the enzyme preparations used and the endpoints measured.

For the enzymes to be effective, they need to reach the duodenum in sufficient quantity. The main obstacle in this process is the low pH in the stomach which can degrade the enzymes before they reach the duodenum. This problem can be solved in 2 ways. One is use of enteric-coated enzyme supplements. The enteric coat protects the enzymes from

Table 18-1

Clinical Response to Therapy—Meta-Analysis

Reference	Duration of Study	Criteria of Response	Response*
Slaff	2 months	Pain score Analgesic usage	11 of 20 (55%)
Isaksson	0.5 month	10-cm visual analog pain scale Analgesic usage	16 of 19 (84%)
Malesci	8 months	10-cm visual analog pain scale Analgesic usage	12 of 22 (55%)
Halgreen	1 month	10-cm linear analog pain scale	9 of 20 (45%)
Mossner	1 month	Pain score (slight, moderate, severe)	25 of 43 (58%)
Larvin	2 months	Pain scale (0 to 5) Analgesic usage	29 of 65 (45%)

*Number of patients obtaining greater pain relief from pancreatic enzymes than from placebo/total sample size (percent).

being degraded in the stomach by the stomach acid. In the duodenum, as the pH goes up the coat dissolves and the enzymes are released. Non-enteric-coated preparations can be efficacious in patients with minor steatorrhea but fail in severe cases. The enzyme release also depends on the particle size. Preparations with particle size of 1.0 to 1.2 mm are more effective than those with particle size of 1.8 to 2.0 mm because the latter release the enzyme more slowly. The other measure to ensure that enzymes are not degraded by stomach acid is to use H2 blockers or proton pump inhibitors (PPIs). Also analgesics like nonsteroidal anti-inflammatory drugs (NSAIDs) can be used to relieve pain. Proteases inactivate lipases. For pain relief, proteases are more important, and for decreasing steatorrhea, lipases are more important. Hence, depending on what is the patient's major problem, you need to decide the balance between these 2 types of enzymes.

Pancreatic enzymes should be taken before the main meals (breakfast, lunch, dinner) and also before the in-between snacks. If a H2 blocker or a PPI is prescribed, then it should be taken about 1 hour before the meal. The enzymes should be taken about half an hour before the meal. The starting dose is about 1 to 3 tablets or capsules of the available enzyme product before each meal. The patient should take about 1 tablet or capsule before the in-between snacks. Each patient should receive individualized enzyme therapy. Different preparations have different enzyme activity. It is not advisable to change or substitute the preparation the patient is using with some other preparation. If for some reason the contents of the capsule need to be mixed, they should be mixed with soft food with pH not less than 5.5. If a patient misses a dose, tell him or her to take it as soon as possible after the meal. However, if the patient is close to the next dose, ask him or her to just continue the regular dosing schedule without double dosing. Although antacids like H2 blockers or PPIs are used as adjuvant therapy, antacids containing calcium carbonate or magnesium hydroxide may interfere with the action of pancreatic enzymes and hence should be avoided.

Adequate diet with appropriate dietary modifications is equally important and would maximize the benefits of the enzyme therapy. Adverse effects of pancreatic enzymes are uncommon. Patients can have hypersensitivity reaction. Nausea, diarrhea, and bloating can occur. However, it is difficult to differentiate this from the symptoms of underlying disease. Some case reports from cystic fibrosis patients have shown colonic strictures with very high doses. The safety of these enzymes in pregnancy has not been studied in humans or animals. They have not been shown to cause problems during breastfeeding.

The main benefit of pancreatic enzyme therapy is to decrease steatorrhea and correct malabsorption. A decrease in steatorrhea can result in preserving the calories from the dietary fat and can help increase or maintain body weight. Certain subgroups of patients like young women and patients with small duct disease benefit more from pancreatic enzyme therapy than others. However, based on the results of our previously published meta-analysis, pancreatic enzymes are not likely to be useful for the management of pain in patients with chronic pancreatitis. It is possible that in select patients with properly administered pancreatic enzyme preparations as discussed, a benefit will be seen. However, it is not clear whether this finding is a true decrease in pain from the medication or a placebo effect.

Bibliography

Brown A, Hughes M, Tenner S, et al. Does pancreatic enzyme supplementation reduce pain in patients with chronic pancreatitis: a meta-analysis. *Am J Gastroenterol.* 1997;92(11):2032-2035.

Bruno M, Haverkort EB, Tytgat GNJ, et al. Maldigestion associated with exocrine pancreatic insufficiency: implications of gastrointestinal physiology and properties of enzyme preparations for a cause-related and patient-tailored treatment. *Am J Gastroenterol.* 1995;90(9):1383-1393.

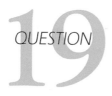
WHAT IS THE PATHOPHYSIOLOGY OF ALCOHOL-INDUCED INJURY TO THE PANCREAS?

Nison Badalov, MD and Scott Tenner, MD, MPH

Alcohol causes at least 30% of cases of acute pancreatitis. Alcohol is the most common etiology of chronic pancreatitis in developed countries. Interestingly, only 10% of chronic alcoholics develop chronic pancreatitis. The classic teaching is that alcohol causes chronic pancreatitis, and that alcoholic patients who present with clinically acute pancreatitis have underlying chronic disease. However, a few patients with alcohol-induced acute pancreatitis by clinical criteria do not have or progress to chronic pancreatitis, even with continued alcohol abuse. By contrast, a small percentage of chronic alcoholic patients develop attacks of acute pancreatitis that are indistinguishable from other forms of acute pancreatitis, but eventually develop chronic pancreatitis after 10 to 20 years of alcohol abuse. Early in the course of the disease, when attacks occur, the diagnosis of underlying chronic pancreatitis is difficult without tissue specimens because the diagnosis of chronic pancreatitis is usually made after definite signs of chronic pancreatitis appear (eg, pancreatic calcification, exocrine and endocrine insufficiency, or typical duct changes by computed tomography [CT], endoscopic ultrasound [EUS], or magnetic resonance or endoscopic retrograde cholangiopancreatography [MRCP or ERCP]). Most of the models described suggest possible mechanisms of alcohol-related injury, including perturbations in exocrine function, changes in cellular lipid metabolism, induction of oxidative stress, and activation of stellate cells. However, the exact mechanism remains unclear and may be related to other factors.

Bordalo and colleagues[1] first proposed that alcohol was directly toxic to the acinar cell through a change in cellular metabolism. Alcohol produces cytoplasmic lipid accumulation within the acinar cells, leading to fatty degeneration, cellular necrosis, and eventual widespread fibrosis. Fatty acid ethyl esters, byproducts of pancreatic ethanol metabolism, may be the key factor in this "toxic-metabolic" change. Bordalo and colleagues[1] suggested that alcohol produces a stepwise progression from fatty accumulation of fibrosis (direct toxic effects on cellular metabolism). The main limitation to this toxic-metabolic theory of alcohol toxicity is the lack of proof of the steatopancreatitis precursor to fibrosis seen in liver disease.

Henri Sarles[2] emphasized the duality of acute and chronic pancreatitis; they were separate diseases with distinct pathogenesis.[3] Whereas acute pancreatitis can be precipitated in patients with gallstones immediately, alcoholism requires years of toxic effects. Alcohol modulates exocrine function to increase the lithogenicity of pancreatic fluid, leading to the formation of protein plugs and stones. Chronic contact of the stones with the ductal cells produces ulceration and scarring, resulting in obstruction, stasis, and further stone formation. Eventually, atrophy and fibrosis develop as a result of this obstructive process. Several studies have provided mechanisms in which alcohol promotes stone formation, including the known recipitation of GP-2 (a Tamms-Horsfall-like protein), increased secretion and viscosity of pancreatic juice, and hypersecretion of enzymes and lactoferrin. In addition, these ethanol-mediated perturbations in pancreatic exocrine function, specific proteins have been implicated in stone formation. Pancreatic stones consist of a calcium carbonate crystalline lattice interspersed within a gel-like matrix formed of multiple fibrillar proteins and polysaccharides.

In contrast to the stone theory, which is based on the de novo development of fibrosis without acute pancreatitis, the necrosis-fibrosis hypothesis envisions the development of fibrosis from recurrent, perhaps subclinical, acute pancreatitis. Inflammation and necrosis from the initial episodes of acute pancreatitis produce scarring in the periductalar areas and scarring leads to obstruction of the ductules leading to stasis within the duct and subsequent stone formation. Support for this theory comes from histopathologic studies that revealed mild perilobular fibrosis in resolving acute pancreatitis, marked fibrosis with ductal distortion occurring later. It is thought that a stepwise progression occurs to fibrosis from recurrent episodes of acute pancreatitis. Support for this theory is seen in a clinical study by Ammann and colleagues.[4] In this study, 254 patients were prospectively followed after the first episode of alcoholic pancreatitis. There was a direct correlation between the frequency and severity of attacks to the rate of progression to chronic pancreatitis.

Recently, the role of stellate cells in pancreatic fibrosis has been characterized. These vitamin A-storing cells have long been known to contribute to hepatic fibrosis. Now, it has been shown that stellate cells are present in the human pancreas and play a similar role in the development of pancreatic fibrosis. When activated, these cells appear capable of synthesizing collagen and fibronectin. In animal models, alcohol and its metabolite acetaldehyde directly activate stellate cells in the pancreas similarly to hepatic stellate cells. Cytokines in the pancreas of a patient with chronic pancreatitis are quite different from a patient with a normal pancreas. Enhanced expression of transforming growth factor beta (TGF-β1), which promotes pancreatic fibrogenesis and other cytokines involved in the process, has been found in patients with chronic pancreatitis.

Whitcomb and colleagues[5] have proposed an interesting hypothesis for chronic pancreatitis which unifies and incorporates recent knowledge in an attempt to reconcile prior theories. Termed the *SAPE hypothesis*, it is best described as follows: in at-risk individuals, the pancreatic acinar cells are stimulated by alcohol. Fibrosis does not occur because a pro-fibrotic cellular infiltrate is not yet present. A sentinel event occurs as trypsinogen is activated. This event results in a massive inflammatory response. Cytokines are then released and work with the activation of stellate cells in the late phase. The attraction and activation of stellate cells sets the stage for the development of fibrosis. If the inciting factors are removed, then the pancreas returns to normal. If the inciting factor, alcohol, is not removed, the acinar cells continue to secrete cytokines in response to the oxidative stress and the stellate cells continue to be activated. This model, using a sentinel event, also represents a time for disease-modifying therapy, when such therapy becomes available.

In summary, although there are multiple models, the exact mechanism in which alcohol causes chronic pancreatitis is not clear. Further study is needed.

References

1. Bordalo O, Gonclaves D, Noronha M, et al. Newer concepts for the pathogenesis of chronic alcoholic pancreatitis. *Am J Gastroenterol.* 1977;68:278-285.
2. Sarles H. Pathogenesis of chronic pancreatitis. *Gut.* 1990;31:629-632.
3. Tenner S, Freedman S. Chronic ethanol administration selectively impairs endocytosis in the rat exocrine pancreas. *Pancreas.* 1998;17(2):127-133.
4. Ammann RW, Muelhaupt B. Progression of alcoholic acute to chronic pancreatitis. *Gut.* 1994;35:552-556.
5. Whitcomb DC, Schneider A. A model for inflammatory disease of the pancreas. *Best Pract Res Clin Gastroenterol.* 2002;16:347-363.

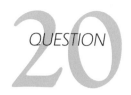

WHEN SHOULD ONE SUSPECT AUTOIMMUNE PANCREATITIS AS A CAUSE OF ACUTE OR CHRONIC PANCREATITIS?

Jonathan Ari Erber, MD and William Franklin Erber, MD

In order to make the diagnosis of autoimmune pancreatitis (AIP), the clinician needs to have a high index of suspicion. Although the classic patient is an elderly male presenting with obstructive jaundice and a pancreatic mass, mimicking pancreatic cancer, the disorder appears to be far more heterogeneous with a myriad of presentations, including pancreatic strictures, fullness to the pancreas, and idiopathic acute pancreatitis.

AIP is a rare form of chronic pancreatitis of presumed autoimmune etiology. Sarles et al[1] first reported pancreatitis associated with hypergammaglobulinemia in 1961, and suggested autoimmunity as the pathogenic mechanism. It is now recognized by many as a systemic autoimmune disorder.[2] The prevalence of this disease has been reported to be 4.6% in Japan, 5.4% in Korea, and 6% in Italy.[3] In the only series reported from the United States, 27 of 254 patients (11%) received a diagnosis of AIP based on histologic findings.[4] Clinical or biochemical autoimmune stigmata are present in 40% of patients with idiopathic pancreatitis.[5]

AIP is seen primarily in elderly males (except when other autoimmune diseases are present), between the ages of 55 and 60. The typical presentation is an elderly male with painless, obstructive jaundice. Diabetes mellitus and impaired exocrine function may be observed. Abdominal pain if present is usually mild. There may be associated weight loss. Patients may also present with typical features of mild, acute recurrent pancreatitis or with biliary and pancreatic duct strictures resembling primary sclerosing cholangitis (PSC). Additional extrapancreatic manifestations include renal (minor renal insufficiency or multiple low attenuation lesions on computed tomography [CT]) and pulmonary (discrete or diffuse nodules, infiltrates, or adenopathy). AIP has also been found to be associated with a number of disorders including PSC, primary biliary cirrhosis, autoimmune hepatitis, Sjogren's syndrome, retroperitoneal fibrosis, inflammatory bowel disease, and antiphospholipid syndrome.[4,6] These associations, however, may in fact be manifesta-

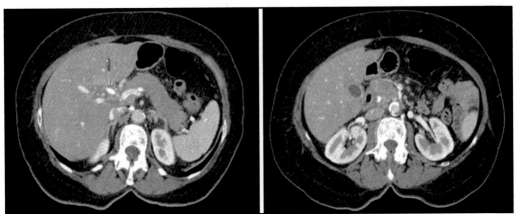

Figure 20-1. Computed tomography image of patient with autoimmune pancreatitis: note relatively large size of pancreas with no mass.

tions of AIP mimicking other well-described diseases and a reflection of a true systemic autoimmune disease.

Diagnosis

A high clinical suspicion is required to make the diagnosis of AIP. The combination of clinical, laboratory, imaging, and histologic findings aids in establishing the diagnosis of AIP and excluding malignancy. The differential diagnosis includes pancreas cancer, alcohol pancreatitis, and idiopathic pancreatitis.

Labs

Hypergammaglobulinemia and elevated serum immunoglobulin G (IgG) levels are detected in about half of patients with AIP. Elevated IgG4 levels are reported to have a high rate of accuracy (97%), sensitivity (95%), and specificity (97%) for differentiating AIP from pancreas cancer.[7] The sensitivity has been reported to be as low as 63% to 68% in other series.[8] A variety of other antibodies, including antinuclear antibody, rheumatoid factor, anticarbonic anhydrase antibody, and antilactoferrin antibody, have also been described to be present in AIP.

Computed Tomography and Magnetic Resonance Imaging

CT and MRI usually demonstrate diffuse enlargement of the pancreas, the so-called "sausage-like" appearance (Figure 20-1).[9,10] Contrast-enhanced CT and MRI will reveal delayed enhancement of the swollen pancreas as well as a capsule-like rim surrounding the pancreas. Focal enlargement of the pancreas may also be seen, similar to that seen in pancreas cancer.

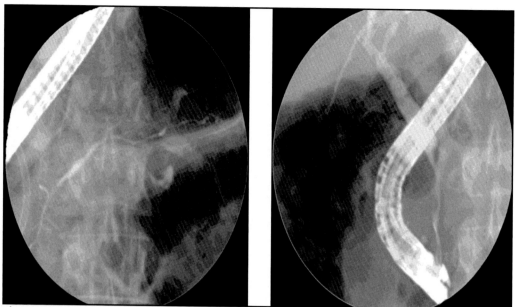

Figure 20-2. Endoscopic retrograde cholangiopancreatography showing stricturing of the pancreatic and bile duct, a double duct sign similar to a malignancy but characteristic of autoimmune pancreatitis.

Endoscopic Retrograde Cholangiopancreatography

ERCP typically demonstrates a diffusely irregular, narrow (<3 mm in diameter) main pancreatic duct (Figure 20-2). In some cases, there is only segmental narrowing of the main pancreatic duct, but the upstream dilatation of the distal pancreatic duct is mild compared to that seen in pancreas cancer.[9] The pancreatic duct may even be normal in appearance. The classic cholangiographic appearance is a distal (intrapancreatic) bile duct stricture. Stenosis of the extrahepatic or intrahepatic bile duct is sometimes observed. The presence of migrating or fleeting strictures that are uncommon in pancreatobiliary diseases other than AIP may be most helpful. Magnetic resonance cholangiopancreatography (MRCP) is less reliable in demonstrating the changes seen on ERCP because it does not adequately visualize the narrow portion of the main pancreatic duct. It does, however, demonstrate stenosis of the bile duct with dilatation of the upper biliary tract.[10] ERCP should be performed in the course of evaluation for AIP when clinically indicated (to provide therapy), not solely to satisfy the diagnostic criteria.

Endoscopic Ultrasound

Characteristic findings with EUS include "sausage-like" pancreatic enlargement with a hypoechoic, coarse, patchy, heterogeneous appearance (Figure 20-3). EUS may also reveal an isolated mass or multiple mass lesions that can mimic "unresectable" ductal carcinoma. Less common EUS features include glandular atrophy, calcification, cystic spaces, features of nonspecific chronic pancreatitis, or even a normal gland.

Figure 20-2. Endoscopic ultrasound of a patient with autoimmune pancreatitis. Hypoechoic image similar to a malignancy.

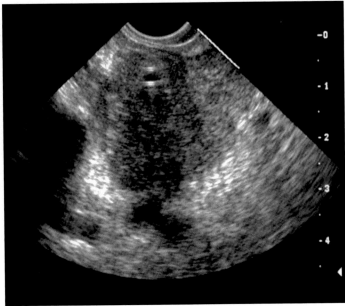

Histology

Obtaining tissue is important in the evaluation of suspected AIP, with the main differential diagnosis being pancreas cancer. EUS with tru-cut biopsy provides core specimens that preserve tissue architecture and permit histologic review.[11] The most common histopathologic findings include fibrosis and an intense inflammatory cell infiltrate comprised mostly of lymphocytes and plasma cells usually surrounding medium- and large-sized interlobular ducts accompanied by an obliterative phlebitis predominantly involving venules. EUS with tru-cut biopsy should be performed when there is a compatible clinical presentation of AIP but in whom there is diagnostic uncertainty and when the findings are likely to alter management. Suggestion that this may be a systemic autoimmune disease is substantiated by the findings of a dense lymphoplasmacytic infiltrate and proliferative myofibroblasts in the gallbladder, bile ducts, kidney, lung, and salivary glands. Focal infiltration of the stomach, duodenum, and colon has been described on endoscopy and confirmed by histology.[12]

Diagnostic criteria have been proposed, both by the Japanese Pancreas Society and the Mayo Clinic group[6,13] (Tables 20-1 and 20-2). The dramatic response to corticosteroids in AIP may be helpful in distinguishing this disease from pancreas cancer and PSC. The majority of patients with AIP will respond to corticosteroids within a few weeks. More recently, several groups have advocated for histology provided by EUS and tru-cut biopsy, along with more liberal imaging criteria to be emphasized in the algorithm for the diagnosis of AIP and in distinguishing between this and pancreas cancer.[11,14]

Table 20-1

Japanese Pancreas Society Criteria for Autoimmune Pancreatitis

1. Typical imaging:
    a. Diffuse pancreatic enlargement
    b. Diffuse (>33%) main pancreatic duct narrowing with an irregular wall
2. Serology: autoantibodies (antinuclear or rheumatoid factor), elevated gammaglobulin or immunoglobulin G
3. Histopathology: lymphoplasmacytic infiltration and pancreatic fibrosis

For the diagnosis of autoimmune pancreatitis, all of the criteria are present or criterion 1 together with either 2 or 3. The presence of imaging criterion is essential for diagnosing autoimmune pancreatitis.[11]

Table 20-2

HISORt Criteria for Autoimmune Pancreatitis

Category	Criteria

A. Histology	1. Diagnostic (any one):
	    a. Pancreatic histology showing periductal lymphoplasmacytic infiltrate with obliterative phlebitis (LPSP)
	    b. Lymphoplasmacytic infiltrate with abundant (>10 cells/hpf) IgG4 positive cells in the pancreas
	2. Supportive (any one):
	    a. Lymphoplasmacytic infiltrate with abundant (>10 cells/hpf) IgG4 positive cells in involved extrapancreatic organ
	    b. Lymphoplasmacytic infiltrate with fibrosis in the pancreas

B. Imaging	Typical imaging features: CT/MR: diffusely enlarged gland with delayed (rim) enhancement ERCP: diffusely irregular, attenuated main pancreatic duct Atypical imaging features: pancreatitis, focal pancreatic mass, focal pancreatic duct stricture, pancreatic atrophy, pancreatic calcification
C. Serology	Elevated serum IgG4 level (normal 8 to 140 mg/dL)
D. Other organ	Hilar/intrahepatic biliary strictures, persistent distal biliary stricture, partotid/lacrimal gland involvement, mediastinal lymphadenopathy, retroperitoneal fibrosis
E. Response to steroid therapy	Resolution/marked improvement of pancreatic/extrapancreatic manifestation with steroid therapy

CT=computed tomography, ERCP=endoscopic retrograde cholangiopancreatography, IgG4=immunoglobulin G4, MR=magnetic resonance.

In summary, the diagnosis of AIP requires a high degree of clinical suspicion. However, it should be remembered that pancreatic cancer is far more common than AIP and a delay in the diagnosis of pancreatic cancer can be devastating. AIP and pancreatic cancer share a very similar presentation, a mass in the pancreas. Failure to establish an early diagnosis of pancreatic cancer may lead to unnecessary morbidity and mortality. An accurate diagnosis of AIP utilizing the appropriate diagnostic and imaging studies illustrated previously may avoid unnecessary laparotomy or pancreatic resection.

References

1. Sarles H, Sarles JC, Muratoren R, et al. Chronic inflammatory sclerosis of the pancreas—an autonomous pancreatic disease? *Am J Dig Dis.* 1961;6:688.
2. Yoshida K, Toki F, Takeuchi T, et al. Chronic pancreatitis caused by an autoimmune abnormality: proposal of the concept of autoimmune pancreatitis. *Dig Dis Sci.* 1995;40:1561.
3. Kim KP, Kim MH, Song MH, et al. Autoimmune chronic pancreatitis. *Am J Gastroenterol.* 2004;99:1605.
4. Pearson RK, Longnecker DS, Chari ST, et al. Controversies in clinical pancreatology: autoimmune pancreatitis, does it exist? *Pancreas.* 2003;27:1.
5. Uzan KN, Levy P, O'Toole D, et al. Is idiopathic chronic pancreatitis an autoimmune disease? *Clinical Gastroenterology and Hepatology.* 2005;3:903.
6. Chari ST, Smyrk TC, Levy MJ, et al. Diagnosis of autoimmune pancreatitis: the Mayo Clinic experience. *Clinical Gastroenterology and Hepatology.* 2006;4:1010.
7. Hamano H, Kawa S, Horiuchi A, et al. High serum IgG4 concentrations in patients with sclerosing pancreatitis. *N Engl J Med.* 2001;344:732.
8. Kamisawa T, Okamoto A, Funata N, et al. Clinicopathological features of autoimmune pancreatitis in relation to elevation of serum IgG4. *Pancreas.* 2005;31:28.
9. Kamisawa T, Egawa N, Nakajima H, et al. Clinical difficulties in the differentiation of autoimmune pancreatitis and pancreatic carcinoma. *Am J Gastroenterol.* 2003;98:2694.
10. Sahani DV, Kalva SP, Farrell J, et al. Autoimmune pancreatitis: imaging features. *Radiology.* 2004;233:345.
11. Levy MJ, Reddy RP, Wiersema MJ, et al. EUS-guided trucut biopsy in establishing autoimmune pancreatitis as the cause of obstructive jaundice. *Gastrointest Endosc.* 2005;61(3):467.
12. Shinji A, Sano K, Hamano H, et al. Autoimmune pancreatitis is closely associated with gastric ulcer presenting with abundant IgG4-bearing plasma cell infiltration. *Gastrointest Endosc.* 2004;59(4):506.
13. Japan Pancreas Society. Diagnostic criteria for autoimmune pancreatitis. *Journal of the Japan Pancreas Society.* 2002;17:585.
14. Nakazawa T, Hirotaka O, Hitoshi S, et al. Difficulty in diagnosing autoimmune pancreatitis by imaging findings. *Gastrointest Endosc.* 2007;65:99.

WHAT ARE THE COMPLICATIONS OF CHRONIC PANCREATITIS?

Jonathan Ari Erber, MD and Frank G. Gress, MD

Chronic pancreatitis can be associated with a variety of complications (Table 21-1). The most common include pseudocyst formation and mechanical obstruction of the duodenum or biliary tree. Other less common complications include external or internal pancreatic fistula with development of ascites or pleural effusion, splenic vein thrombosis, pseudoaneurysm formation, gastrointestinal bleeding, and cancer of the pancreas.

Pseudocysts

Pseudocysts are found in 10% to 25% of patients with chronic pancreatitis and are most commonly seen in patients with alcohol-induced chronic pancreatitis.[1] They are believed to develop as a result of pancreatic duct disruption due to ductal stricturing or intraductal stone formation that occurs from the presence of protein plugs. Pseudocysts may be single or multiple, small or large, and may be located within or even outside the pancreas. They can communicate with the pancreatic duct system and as a result, their fluid usually contains high concentrations of pancreatic enzymes.

PRESENTATION/COMPLICATIONS

Most patients with pseudocysts remain asymptomatic, however, when symptomatic, they can present with a variety of symptoms, signs, and complications depending upon their size and location.[2] Expansion of a pseudocyst may produce abdominal pain, which is the most common presenting symptom. Other less common presenting symptoms and signs include nausea and vomiting (due to outlet obstruction), jaundice (biliary obstruction), and a palpable abdominal mass (cyst expansion). Expansion may also lead to

Table 21-1
Complications of Chronic Pancreatitis

Complication	Signs and Symptoms	Treatment
Pseudocyst	Increased abdominal pain Vomiting Mild elevation in amylase and lipase	Drainage for large or symptomatic pseudocysts: Endoscopic drainage Surgical drainage
Biliary obstruction	Jaundice	Drainage of obstructing pseudocyst Endoscopic decompression Surgical decompression
Gastric outlet obstruction	Abdominal pain Early satiety Nausea and vomiting	Drainage of pseudocyst Surgical gastrojejunostomy
Splenic vein thrombosis	Bleeding from gastric varices	Splenectomy
Pancreatic ascites	Increased abdominal girth High amylase ascites	Endoscopic stent placement Total parenteral nutrition
Pleural effusion	Shortness of breath High amylase pleural fluid	Therapeutic thoracentesis Endoscopic stent placement Total parenteral nutrition
Pancreatic adenocarcinoma	Increased abdominal pain Weight loss	Consider surgical resection Palliation

Adapted from the Cleveland Clinic Disease Management Project: http://clevelandclinicmeded.com/disease management/gastro/chpan/table1.htm.

vascular occlusion, ie, splenic vein thrombosis (discussed below); fistula formation into the adjacent viscera, the pleural space, or pericardium, leading to the development of pancreatic ascites or pleural effusion; and pseudoaneurysms as a consequence of pseudocyst expansion into an adjacent vessel (discussed below). Spontaneous infection and abscess may also occur.

DIAGNOSIS

The combination of persistent abdominal pain and elevated serum amylase and lipase levels can be a clue to the presence of a pseudocyst. The diagnosis is easily confirmed by use of computed tomography (CT).[2,3] We generally perform a contrast-enhanced CT of the abdomen first. CT provides visualization of the pseudocyst's capsule and gauges its maturity. It can also provide the spatial relationship between the pseudocyst and the stomach and duodenum, which is useful in planning interventions such as drainage. Magnetic resonance imaging (MRI) of the abdomen is a reliable alternative to CT.

If a patient is an appropriate candidate for endoscopic drainage, we perform endoscopic retrograde cholangiopancreatography (ERCP) prior to drainage, to identify any ductal obstruction as the underlying etiology and also to identify duct communication with the cyst. Frequently, unsuspected ductal strictures or stones are found, and occasionally a malignant stricture is identified. Magnetic resonance cholangiopancreatography (MRCP) is a noninvasive alternative, but may not be accurate in demonstrating pseudocyst communication as small ducts and fistulas may contain little or no fluid.

Endoscopic ultrasound (EUS) is emerging as an increasingly important tool in the evaluation of pseudocysts.[4] Like CT it provides assistance in localizing the pseudocyst for possible endoscopic drainage and excludes gastric varices, submucosal vessels, and other vascular structures in the pathway of a possible drainage site. Furthermore, it has the additional advantage of providing the opportunity to treat, by performing EUS-guided cystgastrostomy (placing a stent within the cyst for drainage) at the same time. If a linear echoendoscope with a large diameter working channel is used, it is fairly easy and safe to place two or three 10 French stents using only this instrument.[5]

Common Bile Duct Obstruction

Symptomatic common bile duct (CBD) obstruction occurs in up to 10% of patients with chronic pancreatitis. CBD obstruction may result from inflammatory or fibrotic conditions in the head of the pancreas or from pseudocyst compression. Patients may present with abdominal pain and jaundice, with abnormal liver tests, and occasionally cholangitis. We generally perform an MRCP to confirm this diagnosis. We also can perform ERCP if cholangitis is suspected for decompression.

Duodenal Obstruction

Symptomatic duodenal obstruction is seen in about 5% of patients with chronic pancreatitis. The cause is usually fibrosis or an inflammatory mass in the head of the pancreas. Postprandial pain with early satiety is the characteristic presentation, occasionally with nausea, vomiting, and weight loss. Coexistent CBD obstruction may be present as well. The diagnosis is confirmed by CT. Upper endoscopy may underestimate the degree of duodenal stenosis.

Pancreatic Ascites and Pleural Effusion

Pancreatic ascites and pleural effusion may develop as a consequence of pancreatic duct disruption, leading to fistula formation in the abdomen or chest, or from rupture of a pseudocyst with fluid tracking into the peritoneal cavity or pleural space. Patients may present with abdominal distension (ascites) or shortness of breath (pleural effusion). The presence of ascites or a pleural effusion may be obvious from physical exam. Abdominal sonogram and chest X-ray easily confirm the presence of fluid. A diagnostic paracentesis or thoracentesis is diagnostic. Typically, the concentration of amylase in the fluid is very high (>1000 IU/L).

Splenic Vein Thrombosis

The splenic vein courses along the posterior surface of the pancreas, leaving it vulnerable to thrombosis from pancreas inflammation. Splenic vein thrombosis can produce extrahepatic, left-sided portal hypertension and lead to the development of gastric varices in the cardia or fundus. Bleeding is uncommon. If bleeding does occur, splenectomy is curative.

Pseudoaneurysm

Pseudoaneurysms form as a consequence of pseudocyst expansion with pressure and enzymatic digestion of the muscular wall of an artery. Affected vessels are in close proximity to the pancreas and include the splenic, hepatic, gastroduodenal, and pancreaticoduodenal arteries. Their presence is considered rare, but may be seen in up to 21% of patients with chronic pancreatitis who undergo angiography. Bleeding may occur in up to 10% of patients and carries with it a high mortality. The presence of a pseudoaneurysm should be suspected in the setting of patient with pseudocyst who has unexplained gastrointestinal bleeding, unexplained drop in hematocrit, and sudden expansion of a pseudocyst. A CT scan is usually diagnostic. EUS has also been used to diagnose this serious complication. Mesenteric angiography confirms the diagnosis and provides therapy with embolization.

References

1. Yeo CJ, Bastida JA, Lynch-Nyhan A, et al. The natural history of pseudocyts documented by CT. *Surg Gynecol Obstet.* 1990;170:411.
2. Baille J. Pancreatic pseudocysts (part 1). *Gastrointest Endosc.* 2004;59:873.
3. Baille J. Pancreatic pseudocysts (part 2). *Gastrointest Endosc.* 2004;60:105.
4. Chak A. Endosonographic-guided therapy of pancreatic pseudocysts. *Gastrointest Endosc.* 2000;52:S23.
5. Antillon MR, Shah RJ, Steigmann G, Chen YK. Single-step endoscopic ultrasound guided drainage of simple and complicated pseudocyts. *Gastrointest Endosc.* 2006;63:797.

SECTION III

CYSTIC PANCREATIC LESIONS

My Patient Is a Middle-Aged Woman With an Asymptomatic 5-cm Fluid-Filled Cyst in the Tail of the Pancreas, Found Incidentally on Abdominal Computed Tomography Scanning. What to Do Next?

Nison Badalov, MD and Scott Tenner, MD, MPH

Cystic lesions of the pancreas are common. The differential exam is broad and includes benign serous cysts, premalignant mucinous cysts, including intraductal papillary mucinous tumors, cystic pancreatic cancers, lymphoma, and islet cell tumors. Pancreatic cystic lesions are being found with increasing frequency due to more widespread imaging of the abdomen. Most of these cystic lesions of the pancreas are clinically irrelevant and less than 1 cm in size. However, cystic lesions greater than 2 cm in diameter require more attention as they may represent mucin-producing neoplasms. Mucinous cystadenomas (MCNs) typically are found in middle-aged women, are asymptomatic especially when the cyst is less than 5 cm, and are more often found in the tail of the pancreas.

Mucinous cystic neoplasms can become cystic pancreatic mucin-producing carcinomas. These lesions can spread out of the pancreas, rarely become metastatic until later in the course, but can infiltrate locally earlier in the course of the disease. They have a significant mortality rate unless resected. The importance of early resection of the precursor

Figure 22-1. Computed tomography scan demonstrating a mucinous cystic neoplasm causing obstruction of the proximal pancreatic duct in a patient with recurrent acute pancreatitis.

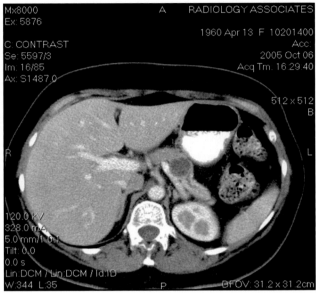

lesions cannot be overemphasized. The slow-growing nature of mucinous neoplasms and their tendency to progress from adenoma to carcinoma, in a sequence similar to colonic adenomatous polyps, provides opportunity to prevent death.

Although the mucinous cystic lesions are noninvasive and easily resectable early, the more diffuse ductal form—intraductal papillary mucinous neoplasms (IPMNs)—are more difficult to resect. Although similar in pathology, differentiating a MCN from an IPMN is important as management differs. Whereas a MCN is loculated and typically focal, IPMNs can be diffuse involving different parts of the pancreas specifically extending through the pancreatic duct. At the time of resection of the lesion, it is important to remove all adenomatous tissue. On endoscopic retrograde pancreatography or magnetic resonance pancreatography, the pancreatic duct is usually not dilated in subjects with MCNs but is typically dilated and containing copious mucin in patients with IPMNs. Only on rare exceptions does the pancreatic duct communicate with MCNs.

For this patient, the issue becomes identification of the mucinous tumor and resection. The differential diagnosis is broad but the important and more common pathology include the need to rule out an IPMN, a serous cystadenoma, cystic solid tumors, and a pseudocyst.

Previous history of acute or chronic pancreatitis should raise the suspicion of a pseudocyst. However, mucinous cystic lesions can cause pancreatitis due to duct obstruction by the cyst or mucin (Figure 22-1). In patients with pancreatitis, previous imaging studies, other evidence of chronicity (eg, dilated duct), and persistence of cyst on follow-up can help determine whether a cystic pancreatic neoplasm caused pancreatitis or whether the cystic lesion is indeed a pseudocyst as a result of pancreatitis.

Cyst fluid analysis (discussed in the next chapter) can also be helpful in the differentiation between MCNs from pseudocysts (Table 22-1). High carcinoembryonic antigen (CEA) values (>200 ng/mL) are nearly diagnostic of a mucinous lesions. However, this level of a CEA has a sensitivity of only about 50%. A low amylase value, less than 250 IU/mL, in the cyst fluid excludes a pseudocyst. However, a high amylase concentration in the cyst fluid does not distinguish pseudocysts from mucinous lesions.

Table 22-1
Cyst Fluid Analysis

Cyst	Viscosity	Amylase	CA 72-4	CEA	CA 15-3
Pseudocyst	Low	High	Low	Low	Low
Serous cystadenoma	Low	Variable	Low	Low	Low
Mucinous cystadenoma	Often high	Variable	Low	High	High
Mucinous cystadenoma carcinoma	High	Variable	High	High	High

It is generally recommended that all mucinous neoplasms of the pancreas undergo resection due to their malignant potential. This advice has been tempered by the marked increase in the number of cystic lesions being identified. Due to their location, distal pancreatectomy is generally the surgery of choice for MCNs. This operation is relatively less morbid than a pancreatic head resection and generally well tolerated. A laparoscopic approach is preferred and typically can be performed with a splenic-preserving approach. Enucleation of the MCN has been reported but not recommended due to high local complication rate and fear of recurrence. Following removal, prognosis is excellent for noninvasive MCN, and recurrence is a rare.

Bibliography

Brugge WR, Lewandrowski K, Lee-Lewandrowski E, et al. The diagnosis of pancreatic cystic neoplasms: a report of the cooperative pancreatic cyst study. *Gastroenterology.* 2004;126:1330-1336.

Chari ST, Yadav D, Smyrk TC, et al. Study of recurrence after surgical resection of intraductal papillary mucinous neoplasm of the pancreas. *Gastroenterology.* 2002;123:1500-1507.

Sarr MG, Carpenter HA, Prabhaker LP, et al. Clinical and pathologic correlation of 84 mucinous cystic neoplasms of the pancreas: can one differentiate benign from malignant and premalignant neoplasms. *Ann Surg.* 2000;231:205-212.

WHAT IS THE BEST APPROACH TO A CYSTIC LESION IN THE TAIL VS HEAD OF THE PANCREAS WHEN THE DIAGNOSIS CANNOT BE CLEARLY ESTABLISHED?

Nison Badalov, MD and Scott Tenner, MD, MPH

Pancreatic cystic lesions are being diagnosed with increasing frequency in asymptomatic patients or incidentally through investigation of an unrelated presenting symptom. With the standard use of cross-sectional imaging, such as computed tomography (CT) or magnetic resonance imaging (MRI), pancreatic cystic lesions are found more commonly than previously reported. Furthermore, through expanding expertise at tertiary care centers as well as in the community setting, endoscopic ultrasound (EUS) evaluation and classification of pancreatic cystic lesions have become possible without the need for surgical extirpation. These imaging modalities allow the treatment algorithm used by most gastroenterologists and pancreatic surgeons to focus on the differentiation of benign cysts from those cysts that are malignant or have malignant potential.

Historically, the majority of fluid collections associated with the pancreas have been classified as pseudocysts or inflammatory in nature. During the evaluation of a patient with a newly diagnosed pancreatic cyst, a history of acute pancreatitis is essential to exclude and therefore virtually eliminate pseudocyst from the differential diagnosis. Beware the radiologist who has little if any historical information and simply writes into the report the finding of a pseudocyst. As diagnostic techniques have expanded, many of these previously misclassified fluid collections are now being appropriately diagnosed as a pancreatic cystic neoplasm. For the remainder of this chapter, we will not focus on pseudocysts or congenital simple cysts of the pancreas. Our goal is to help you differentiate benign from malignant cysts of the pancreas and clarify their management based on anatomical location and malignant potential. Benign cystic neoplasms are called serous

Figure 23-1. Cystic neoplasm in the tail of the pancreas. Laparoscopic approach for distal pancreatectomy not difficult in expert hands.

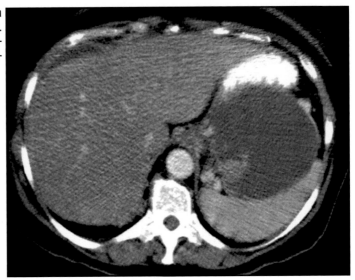

or microcystic cystadenomas. Cysts that are malignant or have premalignant potential are classified as mucinous cystademonas ([MCNs] macrocystic adenoma), mucinous cystadenocarcinoma, side-branch or main duct intraductal papillary mucinous neoplasm (IPMN), solid-pseudopapillary neoplasm, or more rarely a cystic neuroendocrine or cystic ductal adenocarcinoma.

Cysts of the tail of the pancreas are more readily managed with a distal pancreatectomy, spleen-sparing or associated with splenectomy. In carefully selected patients, cysts of the body and tail are able to be removed with laparoscopic distal pancreatectomy, again with or without splenectomy. If symptoms are present, operation should be recommended in the fit patient. Cystic lesions of the pancreatic body or tail that are incidentally found in the asymptomatic patient through investigation of another condition warrant further investigation. For these asymptomatic patients, a minimum of CT and EUS with aspiration should be performed. If characteristics of a mucinous tumor are identified based on imaging characteristics or cyst fluid analysis obtained via EUS aspiration, operation should be recommended. For IMPN, particularly the main-branch variant, margin analysis with intraoperative frozen section is imperative to rule out dysplasia and therefore the appropriate extent of resection. Due to a reported high morbidity rate, we feel that laparoscopic distal pancreatectomy should be an option only at an experienced pancreatic surgery center.

Cysts located in the head of the pancreas are resected with standard or pylorus-preserving pancreaticoduodenectomy (Figure 23-1). Patients presenting with pain or jaundice warrant resection. For the asymptomatic patient, investigation is similar to that for the asymptomatic lesion of the body/tail described above. For patients found to have mucinous cysts of the head of the pancreas, we feel that pylorus preservation provides better gastric function and long-term quality of life without infringing on the oncologic principles of the resection.

For the rare cyst of the neck of the pancreas, a central pancreatectomy may be employed as the procedure for cyst excision. The benefits of central pancreatectomy focus on pancreatic parenchymal preservation. Caution must be used when recommending and performing central pancreatectomy. First, it is of utmost importance to ensure the benign or low-malignant potential nature of the lesion due to the oncologic limitations of central pancreatectomy. Second, several high-volume pancreatic centers have documented a high morbidity rate associated with central pancreatectomy. We feel that only experienced pancreatic surgeons at high-volume centers should be involved in the selection and care of these unique patients.

The decision to operate on a tail or head cyst is multifactorial and must account for patient presenting symptoms, CT and EUS findings, and cyst fluid analysis. We do not necessarily change our diagnostic algorithm based on cyst location alone. At high-volume centers, pancreaticoduodenectomy and distal pancreatectomy are able to be performed with very low morbidity and mortality rates. More importantly, both patient and cyst factors must play a role. Patient fitness must be accounted for but in suitable operative candidates, operative resection should be performed in the symptomatic patient. For borderline candidates or those that are asymptomatic, further investigation to determine the nature of the cystic neoplasm is warranted. CT may reliably differentiate a serous from MCN or IPMN. EUS may be used to evaluate the cystic neoplasm and obtain fluid for cytology, carcinoembryonic antigen (CEA) level analysis, and mucin stain. The presence of mucin or a high CEA level (>192) suggests a mucin-producing or premalignant tumor that warrants resection. EUS also allows evaluation of the cyst wall for the presence of papillary projections or mural nodules, both of which should lead one toward operative excision.

In summary, once a cystic lesion is identified in the pancreas, operative excision should be recommended for the symptomatic patient. In patients who are asymptomatic, further investigation should be performed in order to differentiate a serous (benign) from a mucinous (malignant or premalignant) cystic neoplasm. For mucinous or suspicious cystic lesions, operative excision should be recommended in fit candidates. A team consisting of an experienced pancreatic surgeon, CT radiologist, and pancreatic endoscopic ultrasonographer is critical to completely and appropriately evaluate the increasing number of patients diagnosed with a pancreatic cystic neoplasm.

Bibliography

Baron TH, Adler DG, et al. ASGE guideline: the role of endoscopy in the diagnosis and the management of cystic lesions and inflammatory fluid collections of the pancreas. *Gastrointest Endosc.* 2005;61(3).

Brugge WR, Lewandrowski K, Lee-Lewandrowski E, et al. The diagnosis of pancreatic cystic neoplasms: a report of the cooperative pancreatic cyst study. *Gastroenterology.* 2004;126:1330-1336.

ENDOSCOPIC ULTRASOUND-GUIDED FINE NEEDLE ASPIRATION OF A PANCREATIC CYST IN THIS PATIENT YIELDED FLUID WITH AN AMYLASE OF 4500 AND A CARCINOEMBRYONIC ANTIGEN OF 20. IS THIS NORMAL?

Ilan Aharoni, MD and Scott Tenner, MD, MPH

Pancreatic cysts can vary widely in histology including inflammatory, benign, pre-malignant, and malignant lesions. Since the prognosis as well as the treatment for these lesions is remarkably different depending on the histology, it would be of great clinical benefit to be able to distinguish these cysts in the least invasive way possible.

Often a good history and physical exam may help us to strongly favor one type of cyst over another. For example, one would highly suspect a pseudocyst in the setting of a patient recovering from a recent attack of acute pancreatitis. However, it is often the case that the history and physical are not sufficient to lead us to a definitive diagnosis. Furthermore, with the continuing advances in imaging techniques, we are being referred more and more cases of pancreatic cysts that were incidentally found from imaging modalities done for unrelated reasons. Endoscopic ultrasound (EUS) has become very beneficial for the evaluation of pancreatic cysts. Although the sonographic appearance of pancreatic cysts by EUS may provide us some clues to the underlying histology of the cyst (cluster of microcysts in serous cystadenoma, larger macrocystic structures in mucinous cystadenomas [MCNs]), the sonographic appearance alone is an unreliable marker to

Figure 24-1. Computed tomography showing a pseudocyst. Aspiration of this cyst should show a high amylase greater than 1000 and a low carcinoembryonic antigen.

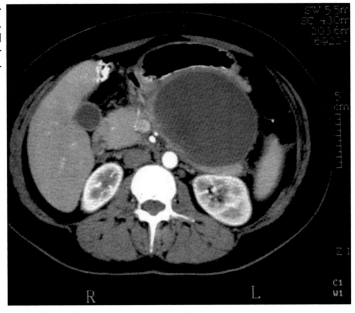

predict histology. Along with the advances in EUS has come needle intervention, which has made sampling pancreatic cystic fluid more available. Even with the possibility of obtaining cytology by fine needle aspiration, there is still a high incidence of false negatives in determining histology. There is a large amount of literature studying the analysis of pancreatic cyst fluid and the utility of this analysis to help predict cyst histology.

For the purpose of this discussion we can break down the various types of pancreatic cysts into four categories: pseudocysts, benign neoplasms (serous cystadenoma), premalignant neoplasms (MCN), and malignant neoplasms (adenocarcinomas). The cystic fluid amylase is helpful to distinguish pseudocysts from the cystic neoplasms. Pseudocysts very often communicate with the pancreatic duct, and therefore usually have very high amylase content of their fluid, usually over 1000 IU/L (Figure 24-1). This concept also applies to ascetic fluid and pleural fluid in patients who may have ascites or pleural effusions related to their pancreatitis. It is important to note, however, that other cystic neoplasms may occasionally communicate with the pancreatic duct as well, and therefore may also have an elevated amylase of their cystic fluid. That is why it remains important to look at your patient in the complete clinical context which would include the history, physical exam, imaging studies, as well as the cystic fluid analysis.

Probably the question of single-most importance when evaluating a pancreatic cyst is whether it is benign or malignant/premalignant. This distinction will have a tremendous impact on the treatment which may involve extensive surgeries with significant morbidities and mortality if the lesion is malignant or premalignant vs a conservative approach for the benign cysts. Various markers of cystic fluid have been studied to assess any correlation with malignant and premalignant lesions. Carcinoembryonic antigen (CEA), CA 19-9, CA 72-4, CA 125, and CA 15-3 are among some of the markers most studied. There are varying results with regard to the ability to differentiate benign lesions from malignant/premalignant neoplasms and to differentiate premalignant from malignant lesions. Most of these studies are of very small sample size. One of the best studies with one of the largest sample sizes studied these various markers to assess any correlation with cyst histology. CEA level of the cyst fluid, with a cut-off level of 192 ng/mL, did show benefit in differentiating mucin-producing cystic lesions from other cystic lesions. In essence, this helps us distinguish between benign lesions and premalignant/malignant lesions.

In summary, it is important to distinguish between different types of pancreatic cysts, even when incidentally found, as they may represent malignant or premalignant neoplasms, which would require more aggressive intervention. Imaging modalities including computed tomography, magnetic resonance imaging, and EUS are not reliable to determine the histology of these lesions. Cystic fluid amylase may be beneficial to diagnose pseudocysts of the pancreas, and positive results are most accurate in the correct clinical context. A high CEA level of the cystic fluid may be beneficial for suggesting a mucin-producing lesion as it has a high specificity, but its lack of sensitivity is important to note, and therefore low levels of cystic fluid CEA should not be used to rule out malignant and premalignant lesions.

It is important to remember that fine needle aspiration of pancreatic lesions, although generally safe, does carry a small but significant risk. Known complications include infection, bleeding, perforation, inducing pancreatitis, and there is the theoretical risk of the seeding of malignant cells when introducing a needle into a malignant lesion. Thus, as in many clinical decisions, you must weigh the risks of the intervention with the benefit of the result. In short, checking the amylase and CEA of pancreatic cystic fluid may be beneficial in some circumstances, but we should only put our patients through the risk of the procedure if the result will change our treatment plan.

Bibliography

Brugge WR, Lewandrowski K, Lee-Lewandrowski E, et al. Diagnosis of pancreatic cystic neoplasms: a report of the cooperative pancreatic cyst study. *Gastroenterology.* 2004;126:1330-1336.

Frossard JL, Amouyal P, Amouyal G, et al. Performance of endosonography-guided fine needle aspiration and biopsy in the diagnosis of pancreatic cystic lesions. *Am J Gastroenterol.* 2003;98:1516.

Hammel P, Levy P, Voitot H, et al. Preoperative cyst fluid analysis is useful for the differential diagnosis of cystic lesions of the pancreas. *Gastroenterology.* 1995;108:1230.

Khalid A, McGrath KM, Zahid M, et al. The role of pancreatic cyst fluid molecular analysis in predicting cyst pathology. *Clinical Gastroenterology and Hepatology.* 2005;3:967.

WHY IS IT IMPORTANT TO DISTINGUISH SEROUS CYSTADENOMA AND MUCINOUS CYSTADENOMA?

Hani Abdallah, MD and Alphonso Brown, MD, MS Clin Epi

Cystic lesions of the pancreas account for 1% to 2% of pancreatic neoplasms. These lesions are increasingly being diagnosed in asymptomatic patients due advances in abdominal imaging with computed tomography (CT) and ultrasound imaging. The most common cystic lesions of the pancreas are mucinous cystadenomas (MCNs) (Figure 25-1), serous cystadenomas (Figure 25-2), and intraductal papillary mucinous tumors (IPMT) (Figure 25-3). These are distinguished from inflammatory pseudocysts in that the last lacks an epithelial lining, septae, loculations, and wall calcifications.

These lesions are more common in women than men and in individuals older than 50 years of age. They tend to be asymptomatic and found incidentally during imaging for other reasons. When symptomatic, they can cause vague abdominal pain or discomfort and a palpable abdominal mass when they attain a large size. Weight loss and obstructive jaundice are uncommon and they point toward a malignant tumor. MCNs are more common than serous cystadenomas. Inflammatory pseudocysts are often preceded with a history of pancreatitis or trauma. Serous cystadenoma have been noted to be associated with von Hippel-Lindau disease.

Once an inflammatory pseudocyst is ruled out, it is important to distinguish those cystic lesions with malignant potential like MCNs and IPMTs from serous cystadenomas. Those tumors with malignant potential may require surgical resection as compared to serous cystadenomas where observation is sufficient (Table 25-1).

Methods to diagnose these tumors are imaging which includes endoscopic ultrasound (EUS) and abdominal CT. EUS has the advantage of allowing fine needle aspiration and cyst fluid analysis for viscosity, amylase, tumor markers like carcinoembryonic antigen (CEA) and CA 72-4 and cytology (Table 25-2). Magnetic resonance imaging (MRI) and magnetic resonance cholangiopancreatography (MRCP) can be used with the advantage of imaging the pancreatic duct with less radiation. The visualization of widely patulous ampulla with mucin extrusion is diagnostic for IPMT.

Figure 25-1. Mucinous cystadenoma on computed tomography: note the cystic lesion in the tail of the pancreas containing solid material, tissue that is perfused.

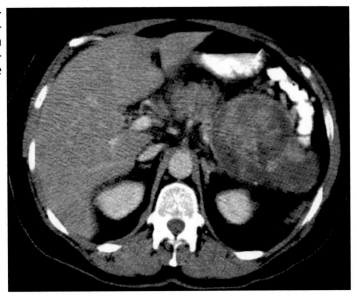

Figure 25-2. Serous cystadenoma on computed tomography: note the clear cyst with a clean wall appearing like a pseudocyst, yet the patient has no history of pancreatitis.

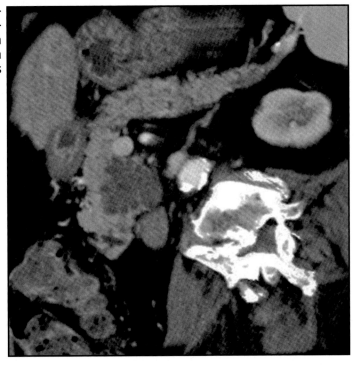

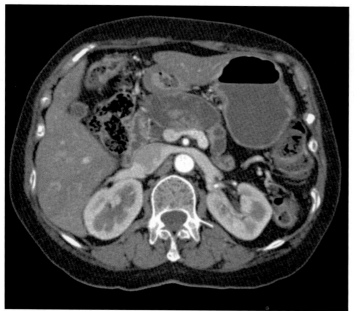

Figure 25-3. Intraductal mucinous papillary tumor on computed tomography: with features similar to a mucinous cystadenoma but the pancreatic duct is involved to the tail with ductal dilatation.

Table 25-1

Clinical Differences Between Cystic Neoplasms of the Pancreas

	Mucinous Cystadenomas	*Serous Cystadenomas*	*Intraductal Papillary Mucinous Tumors*
Sex	Female	Female	Male
Presentation	Pain, mass	Pain, mass	Pancreatitis
Location	Body and tail	Body and tail	Head
CT	Septae, calcification	Septae, calcification (central scar)	Main pancreatic duct or ductal branch involvement
ERCP	Ductal displacement	Ductal displacement	Ductal dilatation, filling defects, duct-cyst communication, patulous ampulla with mucin
Malignent potential	Yes	No	Yes
Treatment	Resection	Observation	Resection

CT=computed tomography, ERCP=endoscopic retrograde cholangiopancreatography.

Table 25-2

Differences in Cyst Fluid Analysis of Pancreatic Cystic Neoplasms

	Pseudocyst	*Serous Cystadenoma*	*Mucinous Cystadenoma (Benign)*	*Mucinous Cystadenoma (Malignant)*
Viscosity	Low	Low	High	High
Amylase	High	Low	Low	Low
CEA	Low	Low	High	High
CA 72-4	Low	Low	Intermediate	High
Cytology	Histiocytes	Negative or cuboidal cells	Mucinous epithelial cells	Adenocarcinoma

In summary, regardless of imaging modality, transabdominal US, CT, or MRI, a cyst in the pancreas may be a benign serous cystadenoma or a potentially malignant MCN. For this reason, multiple diagnostic tests may be needed to determine the exact nature. At times, only surgical resection can clearly establish whether a cyst is serous or mucinous. Although a conservative approach may be reasonable in elderly patients, younger patients should undergo surgical resection if the diagnosis is unclear, especially if the cystic lesion is greater than 2.5 cm. The fear is that a benign, but potentially malignant mucinous cyst will undergo malignant transformation, spread, and become unresectable.

Bibliography

Baron TH, Adler DG, et al. ASGE guideline: the role of endoscopy in the diagnosis and the management of cystic lesions and inflammatory fluid collections of the pancreas. *Gastrointest Endosc.* 2005;61(3).

Brugge WR, Lewandrowski K, Lee-Lewandrowski E, et al. Diagnosis of pancreatic cystic neoplasms: a report of the cooperative pancreatic cyst study. *Gastroenterology.* 2004;126:1330-1336.

Frossard JL, Amouyal P, Amouyal G, et al. Performance of endosonography-guided fine needle aspiration and biopsy in the diagnosis of pancreatic cystic lesions. *Am J Gastroenterol.* 2003;98:1516.

Hammel P, Levy P, Voitot H, et al. Preoperative cyst fluid analysis is useful for the differential diagnosis of cystic lesions of the pancreas. *Gastroenterology.* 1995;108:1230.

Khalid A, McGrath KM, Zahid M, et al. The role of pancreatic cyst fluid molecular analysis in predicting cyst pathology. *Clinical Gastroenterology and Hepatology.* 2005;3:967.

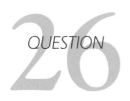

MY HOSPITAL DOES NOT HAVE AN ENDOSCOPIC ULTRASONOGRAPHER. IS IT SAFE FOR ME TO USE COMPUTED TOMOGRAPHY-GUIDED FINE NEEDLE ASPIRATION FOR A PANCREATIC LESION?

Richard O' Farrell, MD

Fine needle aspiration biopsy is a safe and minimally invasive method which may used to obtain a tissue diagnosis of a pancreatic lesion under imaging guidance. Other modalities for obtaining a biopsy of a pancreatic mass include computed tomography (CT), ultrasound, magnetic resonance imaging (MRI)-guided approaches, and, of course, laparoscopy or laparotomy-operative biopsy. Unfortunately, endoscopic ultrasound (EUS)-guided fine needle aspiration is not available at all hospitals.

The specificity of fine needle aspiration biopsy is less than perfect. Put simply, a negative biopsy result cannot be relied upon to exclude cancer. Therefore, the first question to ask oneself and to discuss with the surgeon who is to be involved is "Do we really need to subject the patient to a procedure in order to obtain a preoperative tissue diagnosis?" If there will be no change to management, and an operation will be performed in any event, then it may be reasonable to avoid a fine needle biopsy altogether.

Both CT and EUS have the ability to provide additional information aside from sampling for tissue. Each provides information about stage. EUS is particularly suited to the detection of peripancreatic lymph nodes and can sample them for their involvement. CT excels at defining vascular anatomy and detecting liver metastases of over 1 cm in size. Neither modality reliably detects metastatic deposits on the surface of the liver, or in the peritoneum, which may not be discovered until a laparoscopy.

When facing the choice between EUS as opposed to CT-guided fine needle aspiration biopsy techniques, the deciding factors include the safety and accuracy of the approach, the wishes of the patient, and the availability and expertise of the proceduralists and pathologists involved. The availability of on-site cytological evaluation is desirable. Some studies suggest that the 2 methods are equally effective for lesions both less than and greater than 3 cm.[1-3] Others disagree: 1 retrospective study evaluated 1050 consecutive patients who underwent fine needle aspiration biopsy of the pancreas by ultrasound, CT-guided, or EUS-guided fine needle aspiration biopsies in a single institution. It was found that there was greater accuracy for EUS than ultrasound or CT for lesions less than 3 cm in size.[4]

Whenever I am deciding to send a patient out of hospital for a test elsewhere, I take into account the requirement for excellent and timely communication of the results, the risk of any delay that may be incurred, and finally the cost. Patients who have been informed that they have a mass in the pancreas are understandably anxious to have a firm diagnosis with accurate staging so that they may commence appropriate treatment as soon as possible. In my experience, patients often express concern regarding the risk of rapid tumor progression and may rush to the first available investigation, believing that any procedure is better than a diagnostic delay.

The risks of CT-guided fine needle aspiration biopsy for a pancreatic lesion include bleeding, pancreatitis, vasovagal reaction, tumor seeding, and pancreatic ductal fistula.[5] The approach may be from anterior or from posterior. A coaxial needle may be used to sample even lesions that lie deep to the inferior vena cava or renal vein. Even when major veins, a renal artery, or the gastrointestinal tract is traversed by a needle, the risk of significant hemorrhage and peritonitis (even with transcolonic sampling) is extremely low.[6] Tumor seeding is also an exceptionally rare occurrence.

The risks of EUS need to be taken into account when deciding which modality is best. These include the risks of sedation, perforation, pancreatitis, and bleeding. When using EUS, there are specific anatomic considerations such as ability to pass the scope, prevented, for example, by an esophageal stricture, or the presence of postoperative alterations in anatomy, such as gastric bypass surgery, which may prevent access to lesions in the head of the pancreas.

The efficacy and accuracy of EUS and CT has been assessed in several studies and the results vary.[7,8] Some studies have suggested that the 2 modalities are equally able to safely sample all pancreatic lesions, regardless of size and location. Other studies do not. EUS-guided fine needle aspiration biopsy seems to have the edge for investigation of lesions less than 3 cm and may have advantages when investigating lesions that lie deep to intestine, arterial structures, inferior vena cava, and renal vein when approached under CT guidance.

References

1. Erturk SM, Mortele KJ, Tuncali K, Saltzman JR, Lao R, Silverman SG. Fine-needle aspiration biopsy of solid pancreatic masses: comparison of CT and endoscopic sonography guidance. *American Journal of Roentgenology.* 2006;187:1531-1535.
2. Horwhat JD, Paulson EK, McGrath K, et al. A randomized comparison of EUS-guided FNA versus CT or US-guided FNA for the evaluation of pancreatic mass lesions. *Gastrointest Endosc.* 2006;63:966-975.

3. Mallery JS, Centeno BA, Hahn PF, Chang Y, Warshaw AL, Brugge WR. Pancreatic tissue sampling guided by EUS, CT/US, and surgery: a comparison of sensitivity and specificity. *Gastrointest Endosc.* 2002;56:218-224.
4. Volmar KE, Vollmer RT, Jowell PS, Nelson RC, Xie HB. Pancreatic FNA in 1000 cases: a comparison of imaging modalities. *Gastrointest Endosc.* 2005;61:854-861.
5. Elvin A, Andersson T, Scheibenpflug L, Lindgren PG. Biopsy of the pancreas with a biopsy gun. *Radiology.* 1990;176:677-679.
6. Gupta S, Ahrar K, Morello FA Jr, Wallace MJ, Hicks ME. Masses in or around the pancreatic head: CT-guided coaxial fine-needle aspiration biopsy with a posterior transcaval approach. *Radiology.* 2002;222:63-69.
7. Chaya C, Nealon WH, Bhutani MS. EUS or percutaneous CT/US-guided FNA for suspected pancreatic cancer: when tissue is the issue. *Gastrointest Endosc.* 2006;63:976-978.
8. Brandt KR, Charboneau JW, Stephens DH, Welch TJ, Goellner JR. CT- and US-guided biopsy of the pancreas. *Radiology.* 1993;187:99-104.

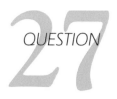
How Does One Manage Pseudocysts?

Nison Badalov, MD and Scott Tenner, MD, MPH

When approached with the patient with a pseudocyst, the first aspect in care requires verification that the lesion is in fact a pseudocyst, defined as a fluid-filled cystic structure in the pancreas or near the pancreas, rich in pancreatic enzymes and surrounded by a fibrous wall of tissue. It is important to remember that radiologists often do not have clinical information on the patient and may inappropriately call a fluid collection or any cystic lesion a pseudocyst. In the absence of a clear history of acute pancreatitis or chronic pancreatitis, a pancreatic cystic lesion will rarely be a pseudocyst. In patients with acute pancreatitis, at least 4 weeks should have passed from admission before a fibrous wall will have formed. Early in the course of acute pancreatitis, calling a fluid collection a pseudocyst is inappropriate. In a patient with no past medical history of chronic pancreatitis who presents with acute pancreatitis and is found on admission to have a cystic lesion that appears to be a pseudocyst, the lesion may very likely be a cystic neoplasm rather than a pseudocyst.

Another important differentiation that is often needed is that of a pseudocyst vs pancreatic necrosis. In a patient with acute pancreatitis, a fluid collection or walled-off cystic lesion in the pancreas often appears and is interpreted by radiologists as being a pseudocyst. However, although cystic fluid in the pancreas has an attenuation on computed tomography (CT) much lower than that of normal pancreatic tissue (Figure 27-1), pancreatic necrosis appears similar. Pancreatic necrosis, especially walled-off pancreatic necrosis (WOPN) (Figure 27-2) cannot be differentiated from a pseudocyst by CT. This is important as the treatment of a symptomatic or infected pseudocyst (abscess) and pancreatic necrosis are quite different. The differentiation between pancreatic necrosis and pseudocysts can often be made by the location of the cyst in relation to the pancreas (Figure 27-3). Whereas pseudocysts are located outside the parenchyma of the pancreas or adjacent, pancreatic necrosis will always involve the pancreas.

Figure 27-1. Pseudocyst. This patient was found to have this fluid-filled, walled-off collection 2 months after an attack of acute pancreatitis. She was unable to tolerate normal meals. After developing post-prandial pain and persistent weight loss, endoscopic drainage was performed.

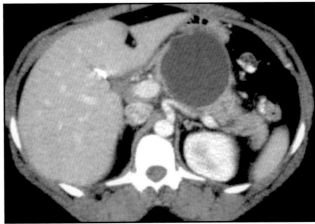

Figure 27-2. Pancreatic necrosis. Two weeks after an admission for acute pancreatitis, this patient developed a fever and was found to have this cystic lesion in the pancreas. Although the radiologist wrote that the patient had a pseudocyst, this lesion is pancreatic necrosis. Drainage, if needed, would require surgical intervention due to the solid components in the cyst.

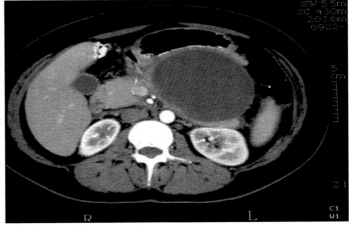

In the past, it became a standard of care that pseudocysts greater than 6 cm or those that are enlarging on serial imaging or become symptomatic warrant drainage. Studies by Mike Sarr[1] and Charles Yeo[2] showed that asymptomatic pseudocysts that may develop after an attack of acute pancreatitis, regardless of size, can be managed conservatively (ie, no intervention). Pseudocysts can become infected, and when this occurs, they are best described as an abscess (abseses require drainage). Pseudocysts can become painful, especially in patients with chronic pancreatitis. Pseudocysts can also cause early satiety and weight loss when their size affects the stomach and bowel. When confronted with a patient who has a symptomatic pseudocyst, whether it is infected or painful, drainage is recommended.

Drainage can be performed via endoscopic, radiologic, or surgical techniques depending on the location of the cyst and the expertise available. No randomized prospective trials have compared these methods. The myriad of size, locations, anatomy, and local expertise make prospective randomized trials difficult.

Surgical drainage of a pseudocyst is possible with a cystgastrostomy or cystduodenostomy if the pseudocyst wall is broadly adherent to the stomach or duodenum. Other procedures include a Roux-en-Y cystjejunostomy or pancreatic resection if the pseudocyst

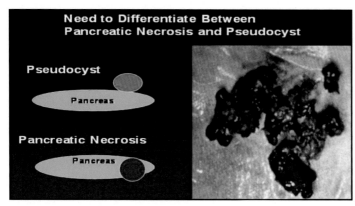

Figure 27-3. There is a need to differentiate pancreatic necrosis from a pseudocyst in patients following an attack of acute pancreatitis. On computed tomography imaging, with or without contrast, the cystic lesions have similar hounsefield units, and attenuation is similar. Whereas patients with pseudocysts have the cyst outside the pancreas, patients with pancreatic necrosis have the cyst within the pancreatic parenchyma. Although the cyst appears fluid filled by computed tomography criteria, the cyst in the pancreatic parenchyma contains debris and often is mostly solid requiring surgical drainage.

is in the tail. Surgical mortality is 6% or less. Pseudocyst recurrence after internal drainage occurs in 15% of cases and is more frequent if the main pancreatic duct is obstructed downstream from the surgical anastomosis. For this reason, a preoperative endoscopic retrograde cholangiopancreatography (ERCP) is usually done to determine whether there is duct obstruction. In this case, a resection of the pseudocyst is preferred.

Percutaneous catheter drainage is an effective treatment to drain and close both sterile and infected pseudocysts. As with surgical drainage, percutaneous catheter drainage may fail if there is obstruction of the main pancreatic duct downstream from the pseudocyst. Therefore, an ERCP is usually done before attempting catheter drainage.

Two endoscopic methods to decompress a pancreatic pseudocyst are (1) an endoscopic cystgastrostomy or cystduodenostomy or (2) transpapillary drainage via insertion of a stent through the ampulla directly into the pancreatic duct and then into the pseudocyst itself. The former method is possible if the pseudocyst is broadly adherent to the wall of the stomach or duodenum. The endoscopist then inserts a double-pigtail stent through the hollow viscus into the cyst. Some endoscopists also insert a transpapillary pancreatic duct stent into the cyst. This is possible if ERCP shows continuity between the pseudocyst and the main pancreatic duct. With either method, the catheter is removed after 3 to 4 weeks if closure of the pseudocyst is seen by CT scan. Failure of radiologic or endoscopic drainage of a pancreatic pseudocyst increases morbidity and prolongs hospitalization. However, most series show long-term resolution with successful endoscopic drainage of pseudocysts.

There are several complications of endoscopic drainage of pseudocysts. The most important is bleeding; the risk of bleeding may be reduced if endoscopic ultrasonography is used to be certain that there are no large vessels in the drainage area. Infection may occur if the double-pigtail catheter becomes occluded. A nasocystic drain to irrigate the cyst may prevent this complication. An endoscopically placed stent in the pancreatic duct may induce ductal changes identical to those of chronic pancreatitis. For this reason, a stent should be removed after several weeks.

If a pseudocyst accompanies considerable pancreatic necrosis, endoscopic and percutaneous catheter drainage should be used very cautiously because neither technique can evacuate the underlying particulate necrotic material, although both are successful in eliminating the fluid of the pseudocyst itself. In this situation, surgical drainage may be preferred because necrotic debris can be retrieved before completing the cyst-enteric anastomosis.

In summary, the first aspect in the evaluation of a pseudocyst is determining whether the cyst is truly a pseudocyst. Although medical therapy is not likely to be beneficial in pseudocyst, drainage is beneficial in patients with symptomatic disease. From multiple case series, it appears that pain, early satiety, and infection will be relieved by drainage of the pseudocyst. There are currently no randomized controlled studies comparing the various minimally invasive approaches in the management of pancreatic pseudocysts. Depending on the available local expertise and technology, intervention should be applied. It remains unclear whether an ERCP is necessary to document communication with the main pancreatic duct in order to attempt a transpapillary approach compared to a transmural approach. Further study will be needed to clarify the best approach to managing pseudocysts complicating chronic pancreatitis. Due to the minimal invasiveness of the approach, and reported safety and success rates in the literature, if expertise is available, an endoscopic approach is preferred.

References

1. Sarr MG. Selected management of pancreatic pseudocysts: operative versus expectant management. *Surgery.* 1992;111:123.
2. Yeo CJ, Bastidas JA, Lynch-Nyhan A, et al. The natural history of pancreatic pseudocysts documented by computed tomography. *Surgery, Gynecology, and Obstetrics.* 1990;170:411.

Bibliography

Neff R. Pancreatic pseudocysts and fluid collections: percutaneous approaches. *Surg Clin North Am.* 2001;81:399-403.

Rosso E, Alexakis N, Ghaneh P, et al. Pancreatic pseudocyst in chronic pancreatitis: endoscopic and surgical treatment. *Dig Surg.* 2003;20:397-406.

Sharma SS, Bhargawa N, Govil A. Endoscopic management of pancreatic pseudocyst: a long-term follow-up. *Endoscopy.* 2002;34:203-207.

Vitas GJ, Sarr MG. Selected management of pancreatic pseudocysts: operative vs expectant management. *Surgery.* 1992;111:123-130.

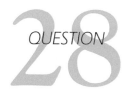

HOW DO I DETERMINE WHEN A PSEUDOCYST HAS BECOME INFECTED? HOW DO I MANAGE THIS?

Nison Badalov, MD and Robin Baradarian, MD, FACG

Pancreatic pseudocyst is a collection of pancreatic secretions enclosed in fibrous tissue layer, without a lining of epithelium. It has continued to be a diagnostic and therapeutic challenge to clinicians. A pseudocyst may occur secondary to acute pancreatitis, pancreatic trauma, or chronic pancreatitis. Pseudocysts complicate 20% to 40% of cases with chronic pancreatitis and 5% to 20% of those with acute pancreatitis. The treatment of pseudocysts includes conservative (medical), radiologic (percutaneous), endoscopic, laparoscopic, and surgical methods. Single pseudocysts are the most common presentation. Multiple pseudocysts are seen in only 5% to 20% of all cases.

Pseudocysts usually contain a high concentration of pancreatic enzymes and variable amounts of tissue debris. Most are sterile. Regardless of size, an asymptomatic pseudocyst does not require treatment. It is satisfactory to monitor the pseudocyst with abdominal ultrasonography every 3 to 6 months. In 2 studies, there was no mortality among patients treated medically or surgically. Pseudocysts can be complicated by infection, intracystic hemorrhage, or rupture leading to pancreatic ascites. Further, pseudocysts can migrate into the chest or other unusual locations. Larger pseudocysts have a higher probability of complications and are therefore more likely to require definitive therapy.

Infection of a pseudocyst occurs in less than 1% of patients. An infected pseudocyst is an abscess and requires drainage. In patients with known pseudocysts, new symptoms, such as abdominal pain, chills, or fever, should alert the clinician to the emergence of an infected pseudocyst or abscess. In the absence of obvious air in the cyst, which denotes infection by gas-producing organisms, imaging cannot distinguish the presence of infection (Figure 28-1). In a patient with a pseudocyst who develops fever, chills, and leukocytosis, suggestive of an infection, drainage is recommended. Establishing infection of the pseudocyst, abscess, is not required. However, computed tomography (CT) is reasonable

Figure 28-1. An infected pseudocyst. There are no signs of infection from imaging.

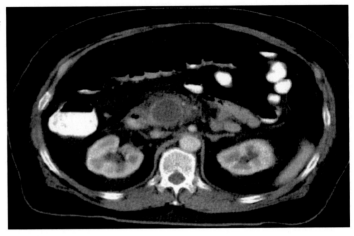

at the time of drain placement. Preoperative endoscopic ultrasound (EUS)-guided fine needle aspiration of cystic lesions of the pancreas is a safe method for determination of the malignant potential, but in a patient with suspected infection and sepsis, performance of EUS with fine needle aspiration, especially under sedation, may be inappropriate.

Treatment choices include surgical, radiologic, and endoscopic drainage. No randomized prospective trials have compared these methods. Surgical drainage of a pseudocyst is possible with a cystgastrostomy or cystduodenostomy if the pseudocyst wall is broadly adherent to the stomach or duodenum. Other procedures include a Roux-en-Y cystjejunostomy or pancreatic resection if the pseudocyst is in the tail. Surgical mortality is 6% or less. Pseudocyst recurrence after internal drainage occurs in 15% of cases and is more frequent if the main pancreatic duct is obstructed downstream from the surgical anastomosis. For this reason, a preoperative endoscopic retrograde cholangiopancreatography (ERCP) is usually done to determine whether there is duct obstruction. In this case, a resection of the pseudocyst is preferred.

The interventional radiologist is often in the position of providing the "last hope" for a patient who has failed standard therapies and is too ill for major surgery. Percutaneous catheter drainage is effective treatment to drain and close both sterile and infected pseudocysts. As with surgical drainage, percutaneous catheter drainage may fail if there is obstruction of the main pancreatic duct downstream from the pseudocyst. Therefore, an ERCP is usually done before attempting catheter drainage.

Two endoscopic methods to decompress a pancreatic pseudocyst are (1) an endoscopic cystgastrostomy or cystduodenostomy (Figure 28-2) or (2) insertion of a stent through the ampulla directly into the pancreatic duct and then into the pseudocyst itself (Figure 28-3). The former method is possible if the pseudocyst is broadly adherent to the wall of the stomach or duodenum. The endoscopist then inserts a double-pigtail stent through the hollow viscus into the cyst. Some endoscopists also insert a transpapillary pancreatic duct stent into the cyst. This is possible if ERCP shows continuity between the pseudocyst and the main pancreatic duct. With either method, the catheter is removed after 3 to 4 weeks if closure of the pseudocyst is seen by CT scan. Failure of radiologic or endoscopic drainage of a pancreatic pseudocyst increases morbidity and prolongs hospitalization. However, most series show long-term resolution with successful endoscopic drainage of pseudocysts.

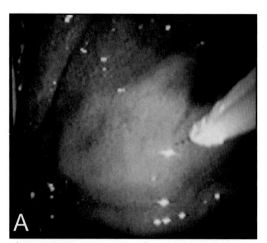 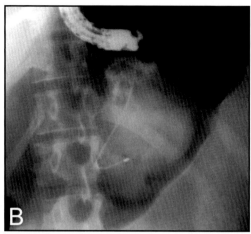

Figure 28-2. Transmural (gastric) approach to drainage of pseudocyst. Note the needle knife (A) and wire placement for stent insertion (B).

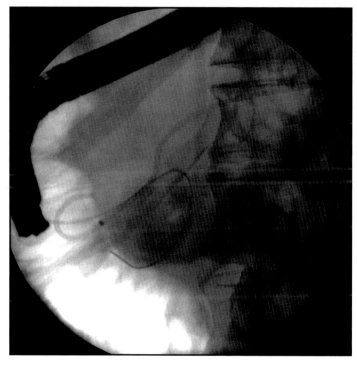

Figure 28-3. Transpapillary drainage of a pseudocyst. Note the wire in the cyst for stent placement.

There are several complications of endoscopic drainage of pseudocysts. The most important is bleeding; the risk of bleeding may be reduced if EUS is used to be certain that there are no large vessels in the drainage area. Infection may occur if the double-pigtail catheter becomes occluded. A nasocystic drain to irrigate the cyst may prevent this complication. An endoscopically placed stent in the pancreatic duct may induce ductal changes identical to those of chronic pancreatitis. For this reason, a stent should be removed after several weeks.

If a pseudocyst accompanies considerable pancreatic necrosis, endoscopic and percutaneous catheter drainage should be used very cautiously because neither technique can evacuate the underlying particulate necrotic material, although both are successful in eliminating the fluid of the pseudocyst itself. In this situation, surgical drainage may be preferred because necrotic debris can be retrieved before completing the cyst-enteric anastomosis.

Multiple pseudocysts pose a unique and difficult therapeutic challenge that has received little attention in the published literature. Unlike single pseudocysts, multiple pseudocysts are less likely to resolve spontaneously and are often more symptomatic. Currently, surgical drainage is considered the treatment modality of choice for multiple pseudocysts.

In the absence of sepsis, and the desire to drain a pseudocyst, there are numerous reports in the literature describing endoscopic drainage (transmural, transpapillary placement of endoprostheses, or both) of single pancreatic pseudocysts. Pancreatic pseudocyst drainage by endoscopy has been employed with increasing frequency; however, the majority of these patients have had simple, uncomplicated pseudocysts. Endoscopic treatment of more complicated pancreatic pseudocysts, including ductal disruption, pancreatic necrosis, or even pancreatic pseudoaneursyms, has been reported previously. Endoscopic treatment of pseudocysts involves transpapillary insertion of a pancreatic duct or a main pancreatic duct stent. In our patients, we prefer to place a main pancreatic duct stent because of the convenience of repeating pancreatograms to demonstrate healing of the duct, without a need to repeat an ERCP. Also, a blocked main pancreatic duct stent can be opened up with flushing and aspiration. This eliminates the need for repeat ERCP and stent placement as in the case of a blocked stent. Once the ductal disruption is healed, the main pancreatic duct stent can be removed without having to repeat an endoscopy. The only concerns with placing a main pancreatic duct stent are the discomfort to the patient and a risk of it being pulled out accidentally.

Regardless of method, drainage of an infected pseudocyst must follow the surgical dictums of adequate drainage, diversion of flow away from and fistula, and adequate antibiotic therapy. Imaging must be performed to assess for drainage. Persistent fluid accumulation likely represents communication with the pancreatic duct and parenchyma. The addition of inhibitors of pancreatic secretion can be considered.

Bibliography

Howell DA, Elton E, Parsons WG. Endoscopic management of pseudocysts of the pancreas. *Gastrointest Endosc Clin N Am.* 1998;8:143-162.

Sharma SS, Bhargawa N, Govil A. Endoscopic management of pancreatic pseudocyst: a long-term follow-up. *Endoscopy.* 2002;34:203-207.

Vitas GJ, Sarr MG. Selected management of pancreatic pseudocysts: operative versus expectant management. *Surgery.* 1992;111:123.

Weltz C, Pappas TN. Pancreatography and the surgical management of pseudocysts. *Gastrointest Endosc Clin N Am.* 1995;5:269.

Yeo CJ, Bastidas JA, Lynch-Nyhan A, et al. The natural history of pancreatic pseudocysts documented by computed tomography. *Surg Gynecol Obstet.* 1990;170:411.

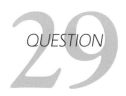
MY PATIENT HAS A LARGE PANCREATIC CYST. SHOULD I INVOLVE A SURGEON IN THE EVALUATION AND MANAGEMENT OF THIS SITUATION?

John D. Christein, MD

Pancreatic cystic lesions are being diagnosed with increasing frequency in asymptomatic patients or incidentally through investigation of an unrelated presenting symptom. With the standard use of cross-sectional imaging, such as computed tomography (CT) or magnetic resonance imaging (MRI), pancreatic cystic lesions are found more commonly than previously reported. Furthermore, through expanding expertise at tertiary care centers as well as in the community setting, endoscopic ultrasound (EUS) evaluation and classification of pancreatic cystic lesions has become possible without the need for surgical extirpation. These imaging modalities allow the treatment algorithm used by most gastroenterologists and pancreatic surgeons to focus on the differentiation of benign cysts from those cysts that are malignant or have malignant potential.

Historically, the majority of fluid collections associated with the pancreas have been classified as pseudocysts or inflammatory in nature. During the evaluation of a patient newly diagnosed with a pancreatic cyst, a history of acute pancreatitis is essential to exclude and therefore virtually eliminate pseudocyst from the differential diagnosis. As diagnostic techniques have expanded, many of these previously misclassified fluid collections are now being appropriately diagnosed as a pancreatic cystic neoplasm. For the remainder of this chapter, I will not focus on pseudocysts or congenital simple cysts of the pancreas. My goal is to help you differentiate benign from malignant cysts of the pan-

Figure 29-1. Pancreatic tail cyst as seen through the mesentery.

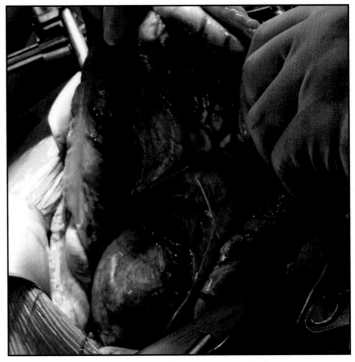

creas and clarify their management based on anatomical location and malignant potential. Benign cystic neoplasms are called serous or microcystic cystadenomas. Cysts that are malignant or have premalignant potential are classified as mucinous cystadenomas ([MCNs] macrocystic adenoma), mucinous cystadenocarcinoma, side-branch or main duct intraductal papillary mucinous neoplasm (IPMN), solid-pseudopapillary neoplasm, or more rarely a cystic neuroendocrine or cystic ductal adenocarcinoma.

Cysts of the tail of the pancreas are able to be managed with distal pancreatectomy, spleen-sparing or associated with splenectomy (Figure 29-1). In carefully selected patients, cysts of the body and tail are able to be removed with laparoscopic distal pancreatectomy, again with or without splenectomy (Figure 29-2). If symptoms are present, operation should be recommended in the fit patient. Cystic lesions of the pancreatic body or tail that are incidentally found in the asymptomatic patient through investigation of another condition warrant further investigation. For these asymptomatic patients, a minimum of CT and EUS with aspiration should be performed. If characteristics of a mucinous tumor are identified based on imaging characteristics or cyst fluid analysis obtained via EUS aspiration, operation should be recommended. For IMPN, particularly the main-branch variant, margin analysis with intraoperative frozen section is imperative to rule out dysplasia and therefore the appropriate extent of resection. Due to a reported high morbidity rate, I feel that laparoscopic distal pancreatectomy should be an option only at an experienced pancreatic surgery center.

Cysts located in the head of the pancreas are resected with standard or pylorus-preserving pancreaticoduodenectomy. Patients presenting with pain or jaundice warrant resection. For the asymptomatic patient, investigation is similar to that for the asymptomatic lesion of the body/tail described above. For patients found to have mucinous

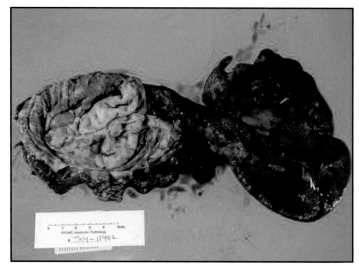

Figure 29-2. Specimen of resection leading to splenectomy due to infiltration of the splenic vein by the cystic mass.

cysts of the head of the pancreas, I feel that pylorus preservation provides better gastric function and long-term quality of life without infringing on the oncologic principles of the resection.

For the rare cyst of the neck of the pancreas, a central pancreatectomy may be employed as the procedure for cyst excision. The benefits of central pancreatectomy focus on pancreatic parenchymal preservation. Caution must be used when recommending and performing central pancreatectomy. First, it is of utmost importance to ensure the benign or low malignant potential nature of the lesion due to the oncologic limitations of central pancreatectomy. Second, several high-volume pancreatic centers have documented a high morbidity rate associated with central pancreatectomy. I feel that only experienced pancreatic surgeons at high-volume centers should be involved in the selection and care of these unique patients.

The decision to operate on a tail or head cyst is multifactorial and must account for patient-presenting symptoms, CT and EUS findings, and cyst fluid analysis. In my mind, I do not necessarily change my diagnostic algorithm based on cyst location alone. At high-volume centers, pancreaticoduodenectomy and distal pancreatectomy are able to be performed with very low morbidity and mortality rates. More importantly, both patient and cyst factors must play a role. Patient fitness must be accounted for but in suitable operative candidates, operative resection should be performed in the symptomatic patient. For borderline candidates or those that are asymptomatic, further investigation to determine the nature of the cystic neoplasm is warranted. CT may reliably differentiate a serous from MCN or IPMN. EUS may be used to evaluate the cystic neoplasm and obtain fluid for cytology, carcinoembryonic antigen (CEA) level analysis, and mucin stain. The presence of mucin or a high CEA level (>192) suggests a mucin-producing or premalignant tumor that warrants resection. EUS also allows evaluation of the cyst wall for the presence of papillary projections or mural nodules, both of which should lead one toward operative excision.

In summary, once a cystic lesion is identified in the pancreas, operative excision should be recommended for the symptomatic patient. In patients who are asymptomatic, further investigation should be performed in order to differentiate a serous (benign) from a mucinous (malignant or premalignant) cystic neoplasm. For mucinous or suspicious cystic lesions, operative excision should be recommended in fit candidates. A team consisting of an experienced pancreatic surgeon, CT radiologist, and pancreatic endoscopic ultrasonographer is critical to completely and appropriately evaluate the increasing number of patients diagnosed with a pancreatic cystic neoplasm.

Bibliography

Baron TH, Adler DG, et al. ASGE guideline: the role of endoscopy in the diagnosis and the management of cystic lesions and inflammatory fluid collections of the pancreas. *Gastrointest Endosc.* 2005;61(3).

Brugge WR, Lewandrowski K, et al. The diagnosis of pancreatic cystic neoplasms: a report of the cooperative pancreatic cyst study. *Gastroenterology.* 2004;126:1330-1336.

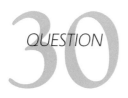
WHEN SHOULD ENDOSCOPIC THERAPY OF THE PSEUDOCYST AND/OR ORGANIZED NECROSIS IN ACUTE PANCREATITIS BE APPLIED?

Nison Badalov, MD and Robin Baradarian, MD, FACG

It is important to use precise terms in describing the anatomic complications of acute pancreatitis. The ability to apply appropriate therapy depends on a clear understanding of these terms. An old term that should never be used in describing these complications is *phlegmon*. This term is unclear and has carried different meaning to gastroenterologists, internists, radiologists, and surgeons. Whereas patients with interstitial pancreatitis (Figure 30-1) have a normally perfused, normally attenuated gland on contrast-enhanced computed tomography (CT), patients with necrotizing pancreatitis (Figure 30-2) have greater than 30% of the gland not perfused, with low attenuation. Pancreatic necrosis consists of focal or diffuse nonviable pancreatic parenchyma and usually peripancreatic fat necrosis. Pancreatic necrosis can be infected or sterile. An acute fluid collection (Figure 30-3) is fluid located in or near the pancreas that lacks a definite wall and that occurs early in the course of acute pancreatitis. On CT scan it is a low attenuation mass with poor margins and no capsule. Intrapancreatic fluid collections are less than 3 cm. An acute fluid collection occurs in 30% to 50% of acute pancreatitis and most resolve spontaneously. A pseudocyst (Figure 30-4) is a fluid collection that persists for 4 to 6 weeks and becomes encapsulated by a wall of fibrous or granulation tissue. A pancreatic abscess is a circumscribed intra-abdominal collection of pus after an episode of acute pancreatitis or pancreatic trauma. It usually develops close to the pancreas and contains little pancreatic necrosis. Due to confusion of whether an abscess represents an infected pseudocyst or infected pancreatic necrosis, the term should be used sparingly. It is best to use the terms *infected pseudocyst* and *infected necrosis*. *Hemorrhagic pancreatitis* should not be used as a synonym for *necrotizing pancreatitis*. This term should also be used with caution.

Figure 30-1. Patient with acute interstitial pancreatitis.

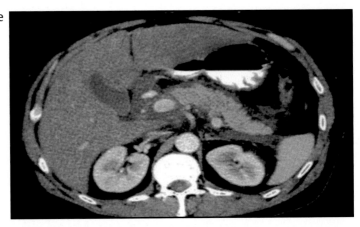

Figure 30-2. Patient with acute necrotizing pancreatitis.

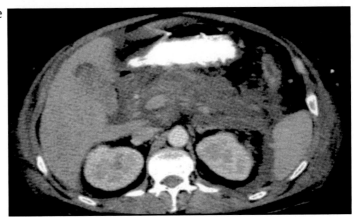

Figure 30-3. Patient with acute pancreatitis and acute fluid collection.

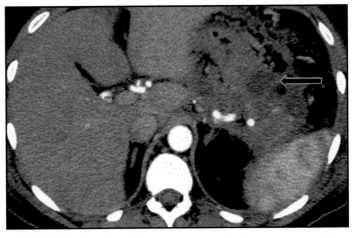

Over the past decade, a new term has emerged, *walled-off pancreatic necrosis* (WOPN) (Figure 30-5). Largely due to advances in minimally invasive surgery, radiology, and endoscopy, this term is used to describe pancreatic necrosis that has liquefied, after 5 to

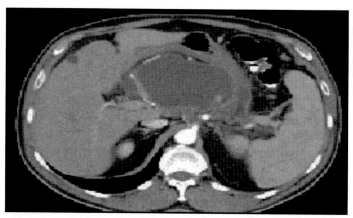

Figure 30-4. Computed tomography of a pseudocyst in a patient presenting with abdominal pain and early satiety 6 weeks following an episode of acute pancreatitis.

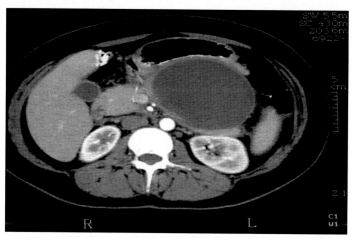

Figure 30-5. Computed tomography of a walled-off pancreatic necrosis in a patient with persistent abdominal pain and anorexia.

6 weeks. Similar to a pseudocyst, a wall develops. However, whereas a pseudocyst always contained fluid, pancreatic necrosis, even if walled-off early, contains a significant amount of debris which only becomes liquefied after 5 to 6 weeks. No attempt should be made to drain WOPN endoscopically or radiologically early (<4 weeks) as the debris is typically thick, often with the consistency of rubber early in the course of the disease. After 5 to 6 weeks, a WOPN can be treated similar to the fluid-filled pseudocyst, drained surgically, endoscopically (Figure 30-6), or radiologically.

Approximately one-third of patients with necrotizing pancreatitis develop infected necrosis. The infection usually occurs after 10 to 14 days of illness. Most patients with infected necrosis have systemic toxicity, such as fever and leukocytosis. Almost half of the patients with infected necrosis have persistent organ failure. The distinction between sterile and infected necrosis is important typically in the second or third weeks when surgical intervention is feasible. The technique of percutaneous CT-guided fine needle aspiration has been shown to be safe and effective. A gram stain of the peripancreatic bed that is carefully observed can lead to a diagnosis in most cases; cultures should be considered confirmatory.

The standard of care for infected pancreatic necrosis is surgical debridement. Currently, there is controversy in the surgical literature regarding the time of surgery. Although

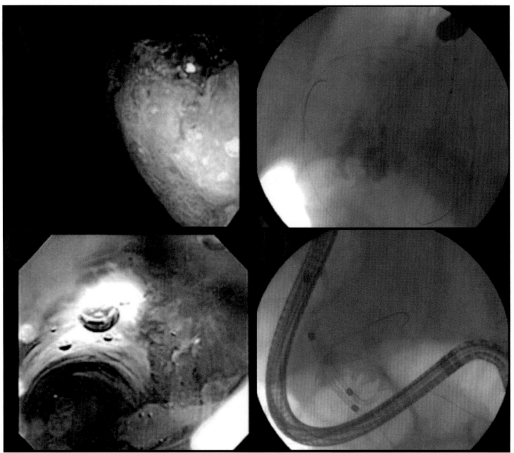

Figure 30-6. Endoscopic transmural drainage of a walled-off pancreatic necrosis. The technique involves the endoscopic identification of the area of maximum bulge (A) with the use of a side-viewing endoscope. Needle puncture and entry into cavity and verification of entry by insertion of guidewire (B) and contrast injection. Balloon dilatation of the needle tract (C) followed by several 7 to 10 French stents insertion (D). These steps may be required to be repeated multiple times for complete resolution of the necrosis.

urgent surgical intervention was the consensus years prior, some authors have now suggested that a prolonged period of antibiotics be given prior to surgery to allow the inflammatory reaction to subside. In addition, several novel techniques, minimally invasive endoscopic and radiologic techniques, have been described to debride infected necrosis. There are also several published reports of patients with infected necrosis undergoing successful treatment with intravenous antibiotics without any surgical, endoscopic, or radiologic intervention. Given the controversy, each case of infected necrosis must be considered individually. The timing of surgical intervention should be determined by the pancreatic surgeon.

Bibliography

Aghdassi A, Mayerle J, Kraft M, Sielenkamper AW, Heidecke CD, Lerch MM. Diagnosis and treatment of pancreatic pseudocysts in chronic pancreatitis. *Pancreas.* 2008;36:105-112.

Baron TH, Harewood GC, Morgan DE, et al. Outcome differences after endoscopic drainage of pancreatic necrosis, acute pancreatic pseudocysts, and chronic pancreatic pseudocysts. *Gastrointest Endosc.* 2002;56:7-17.

Bhattacharya D, Ammori BJ. Minimally invasive approaches to the management of pancreatic pseudocysts. *Surg Laparosc Endosc Percutan Tech.* 2003;13:141-148.

Bradley EL, Clements J, Gonzales A. The natural history of pancreatic pseudocysts: a unified concept of management. *Am J Surg.* 1979;137:135-141.

Brugge WR. Approaches to the drainage of pancreatic pseudocysts. *Current Opinion in Gastroenterology.* 2004;20:488-492.

Brugge WR, Lewandrowski K, Lee-Lewandrowski E, et al. Diagnosis of pancreatic cystic neoplasms: a report of the cooperative pancreatic cyst study. *Gastroenterology.* 2005;126:1330-1336.

Catalano MF, Geenen JE, Schmalz MJ, et al. Treatment of pancreatic pseudocysts with ductal communication by transpapillary pancreatic duct endoprosthesis. *Gastrointest Endosc.* 1995;42:214-218.

De Palma GD, Galloro G, Puzziello A, et al. Endoscopic drainage of pancreatic pseudocysts: a long-term follow-up study of 49 patients. *Hepatogastroenterology.* 2002;49:1113-1115.

Gumaste V, Pitchumoni CS. Pancreatic pseudocyst. *Gastroenterologist.* 1996;433-443.

Pitchumoni CS, Agarwal N. Pancreatic pseudocysts: when and how should drainage be performed. *Gastroenterol Clin North Am.* 1999;28:610-645.

Schlosser W, Siech M, Beger HG. Pseudocyst treatment in chronic pancreatitis—surgical treatment of the underlying disease increases the long term success. *Dig Surg.* 2005;22:340-345.

Usatoff V, Brancatisano R, Williamson RC. Operative treatment of pseudocysts in patients with chronic pancreatitis. *Br J Surg.* 2000;87:1494-1499.

Warshaw AL. Pancreatic cysts and pseudocysts: new rules for a new game. *Br J Surg.* 1988;76:533-534.

Warshaw AL, Rattner DW. Timing of surgical drainage for pancreatic pseudocyst. Clinical and chemical criteria. *Ann Surg.* 1985;202:720-724.

SECTION IV

PANCREATIC CANCER

WHAT ARE THE RISK FACTORS FOR THE DEVELOPMENT OF PANCREATIC CANCER?

Nison Badalov, MD and Robin Baradarian, MD, FACG

In the United States, approximately 30,000 patients are diagnosed annually with pancreatic cancer. There is a wide international variation in the incidence of pancreatic cancer, with incidence ranging from 0.05% to 1%, with highest incidence being found in African-Americans and in the developed, industrialized countries. Although pancreatic cancer represents only 2% of all new cancer cases, it leads to 5% of all cancer deaths.

Despite being a very rare type of cancer when compared to breast and colon cancers, pancreatic cancer ranks fourth as a cause of death from cancer. Most of the patients die within 1 year of diagnosis and have a median survival of 4 to 6 months. Five-year survival rate is less then 5%, with higher rates of survival seen in the minority of patients who are resectable at the time of diagnosis and are candidates for chemotherapy.

Age

Age is one of the most important factors in the development of pancreatic cancer. Incidence of pancreatic cancer sharply rises after age 60, with highest incidence in 7th and 8th decades of life, and average age of diagnosis of 60 to 65 years. Pancreatic cancer can occur in patients at younger ages with strong family history of pancreatic cancer.

Chronic Pancreatitis

Chronic pancreatitis usually results from recurrent attacks of acute pancreatitis that eventually results in the loss of function, development of chronic abdominal pain, and increased risk of pancreatic cancer. Causes of acute pancreatitis can be acquired or inherited. Acquired risk factors for acute pancreatitis include alcohol, gallstones, endoscopic retrograde cholangiopancreatography (ERCP), tropical pancreatitis (seen in parts of India and Africa), drugs, trauma, hypercalcemia, hypertriglyceridemia, toxic-metabolic, etc. Inherited risk factors for acute pancratitis include hereditary chronic pancreatitis (PRSS1/cationic trypsinogen gene mutation), cystic fibrosis (CFTR gene mutation), and mutations in the pancreatic secretory trypsin inhibitor gene (PSTI or SPINK1). Patients with chronic hereditary pancreatitis have the highest lifetime risk of all causes of developing pancreatic cancer—40%.

Diabetes Mellitus

Greater than 80% of patients with pancreatic cancer have diabetes mellitus II or impaired glucose metabolism. It is hypothesized that tumor cells secrete islet amyloid peptide that reduced insulin sensitivity. Resection of tumor improves underlying diabetes and glucose intolerance. A meta-analysis of 20 studies estimated relative risk of 2.1 when comparing diabetics to nondiabetics in the development of pancreatic cancer. In addition, patients who were diagnosed with diabetes mellitus II within the past 4 years had 50% greater chance of development of pancreatic cancer when compared to the patients that were diagnosed with diabetes mellitus II more than 5 years ago.

Diet

Although there is some evidence in the literature that diets rich in fats, calories, and nitrites-preservatives increase the risk of developing pancreatic cancer, human studies have been inconclusive. However, some animal studies showed that diets poor in calories have reduced the frequency of premalignant pancreatic lesions. In addition, some studies reported protective effect of fresh fruits and vegetables against the development of pancreatic cancer.

Conflicting results have been published and failed to demonstrate a relationship between coffee and alcohol consumption and the development of pancreatic cancer. Similarly, large cohort studies failed to demonstrate any protective link between pancreatic cancer and aspirin/nonsteroidal anti-inflammatory drug use.

Gender and Race

Males have a higher chance of developing pancreatic cancer than females. Native Hawaiians, Maori, and blacks have the highest incidence of pancreatic cancer, while Nigerians and Indians have the lowest.

H. pylori is a known carcinogen, implicated in causing gastric cancer. In addition to gastric cancer, H. pylori infection has also been associated with increased risk for the development of pancreatic cancer. The underlying mechanism is thought to be related to hyperacidity, and CagA strains seemed to have the greatest risk.

Obesity

A body mass index (BMI) of 30 kg/m^2 was associated with a definite increase in rate of pancreatic cancer development when compared to BMI of 23 kg/m^2 or less. Physical activity showed inverse relationship to the development of pancreatic cancer.

Partial Gastrectomy

A history of partial gastrectomy leads to 2 to 5 times increased chance of developing pancreatic cancer about 15 to 20 years after surgery. Similar but conflicting results have also been reported in patients with prior history of cholecystectomy.

Smoking

Smoking is a major risk factor to the development of pancreatic cancer. It has been estimated that roughly 25% of pancreatic cancer deaths can be prevented by smoking cessation. Aromatic amines that are found in the smoke are thought to be the carcinogens related to the development of pancreatic cancer. Studies have shown that smoking doubles the risk of developing of pancreatic cancer, and higher rates of pancreatic cancer have been reported in patients who had heavier/longer smoking history. Smoking cessation reduces the risk of developing of pancreatic cancer, however, risk persists for more than 10 years.

In addition to smoking, patients exposed to chemicals such as nickel, chromium, silica, organic solvents, organochlorine insecticides, pesticides, petrochemical, and rubber industries and hairdressers have a slight greater risk of developing pancreatic cancer.

Familial Pancreatic Cancer

Familial pancreatic cancer is rare and accounts for up to 3% of pancreatic ductal adenocarcinoma. It is usually diagnosed when 2 or more first-degree relatives are diagnosed with pancreatic adenocarcinoma and other known risk factors for pancreatic cancer are absent. Although the gene mutation has not been identified yet, there seems to be an autosomal dominant mode of transmission.

Nonpancreatic Cancer Syndromes

There are several nonpancreatic cancer syndromes that increase the risk of developing exocrine pancreatic cancer and include ataxia-telangiectasia, familial adenomatous polyposis, familial atypical multiple mole melanoma, familial ovarian and breast cancer, Fanconi anemia, hereditary nonpolyposis colorectal cancer, Li-Fraumeni syndrome, and Peutz-Jeghers syndrome.

Ataxia-telangiectasia is a condition associated with cerebellar ataxia, oculocutaneous arteriovenous malformations, and defects in the immune system. Several studies have shown an association with increased risk of developing pancreatic cancer.

Familial adenomatous polyposis is a condition in which affected individuals develop numerous adenomatous polyps throughout the colon, which have the potential for malignant transformation. In addition to having a very high risk of developing of colon cancer, there has been some evidence to suggest that these patients may also have increased risk of developing pancreatic cancer.

Familial atypical multiple mole melanoma is a condition that is associated with multiple dysplastic nevi, malignant melanomas, extracutaneous malignancies, and pancreatic cancer. It seems that in patients with familial atypical multiple mole melanoma, mutations in tumor suppressor gene INK4αp16 are responsible for the development of pancreatic cancer. These patients have 17% lifetime risk of developing pancreatic cancer.

Germline mutations in BRCA1 and BRCA2 genes, which are DNA repair genes, lead to the development of familial ovarian and breast cancer syndromes. Several studies showed relative risk of pancreatic cancer in patients with BRCA1 gene mutation to be increased by 2.7 times. Approximately 5% of patients with known BRCA2 mutation will develop pancreatic cancer over their lifetimes, and it is BRCA2 gene mutation that is found in the patients with Fanconi anemia, who also have increased risk of development of pancreatic cancer.

Hereditary nonpolyposis colorectal cancer, also known as Lynch syndrome, results from mutation of several DNA mismatch repair genes. The syndrome is characterized by early development of colorectal, breast, ovary, endometrial, bladder, small bowel, and pancreatic malignancies.

Li-Fraumeni syndrome is a rare condition, characterized by mutation in the Tp53, which is a tumor suppressor gene. Tp53 is found in three-fourths of patients with ductal adenocarcinoma of the pancreas.

Peutz-Jeghers syndrome is a condition that manifests itself by the development of hamartomous polyps throughout the gastrointestinal tract and mucocutaneous pigmentation. Patients with Peutz-Jeghers syndrome have STK11/LKB1 gene mutation and 36% lifetime risk of developing pancreatic cancer.

In summary, although there are many associations with pancreatic cancer, age and smoking are the most common and important risk factors. A history of chronic pancreatitis, related to alcohol or family (cationic trypsinogen), are also important risk factors.

Bibliography

Castillo CF, Jimenez RE. Risk factors for and molecular pathogenesis of pancreatic cancer. UptoDate. www.utdol. com/utd/store/index.do.

Lowenfelds AB, Maisonneuve P. Risk factors for pancreatic cancer. *J Cell Biochem.* 2005;95:649-656.

Vitone LJ, Greenhalf W, McFaul CD, Ghaneh P, Neoptolemos JP. The inherited genetics of pancreatic cancer and prospects for secondary screening. *Best Pract Res Clin Gastroenterol.* 2006;20(2):253-283.

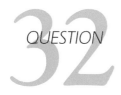
WHAT IS THE BEST APPROACH TO STAGING PANCREATIC CANCER?

Nison Badalov, MD and Robin Baradarian, MD, FACG

Due to the often late stage of diagnosis, pancreatic cancer remains a dreadful disease. Survival and treatment are directly related to the stage of the disease. Although direct laparotomy provides the best method of staging, noninvasive or minimally invasive imaging techniques are preferred. Computed tomography (CT) remains the most accepted first step in imaging to detect advanced disease. However, magnetic resonance imaging (MRI) should be considered equally specific and perhaps more sensitive. Detection of metastatic disease by CT precludes any need for local staging. If a CT or MRI suggests the absence of metastatic disease, endoscopic ultrasound (EUS) is the most accurate method for staging of the local extent of disease (Figures 32-1 and 32-2).

Mass Lesion in a Patient Who Is Unfit for a Major Pancreatic Resection

For patients who are unfit to undergo a major resection, a tissue diagnosis should be made to permit palliation by endoscopic, chemotherapeutic, or radiotherapeutic means. This can be accomplished either by percutaneous (CT- or US-guided) fine needle aspiration biopsy or by endoscopically obtained brushings or biopsies. Endoscopic biopsy can frequently be aided by EUS guidance.

Figure 32-1. Endoscopic ultrasound fine needle aspiration of a suspected early pancreatic cancer.

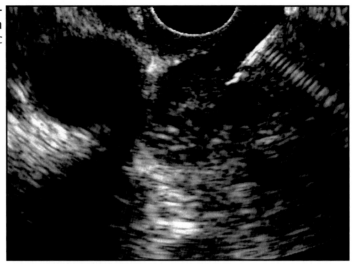

Figure 32-2. Cytology from endoscopic ultrasound fine needle aspiration showing adenocarcinoma.

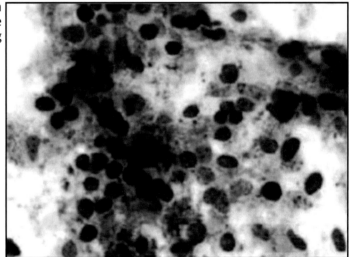

Mass Lesion Not Seen on Computed Tomography or Ultrasound

When no mass lesion is detected on CT or US, an endoscopic retrograde cholangiopancreatography (ERCP) should be performed to exclude biliary tract stones or some other non-neoplastic cause of symptoms. The ERCP may also confirm the suspected diagnosis of pancreatic tumor if a peri-ampullary mass is detected or if malignant-appearing strictures of the pancreatic and/or bile duct are found.

Mass Lesion in a Candidate for Major Pancreatic Resection

When a mass lesion of the pancreas is detected on CT or US, it is reasonable to conclude that a neoplasm (most likely malignant) is present and no further diagnostic tests are needed for patients who are otherwise fit to undergo a major pancreatic resection. Attempts to make a tissue diagnosis in such patients are not useful since a benign sample does not exclude the presence of a neighboring malignancy and, in the absence of a diagnostic sample, one must assume that the lesion is malignant.

Determining Resectability

The next issue for patients who have a mass lesion and who are surgical candidates is determining resectability. Most surgeons limit radical resections to the management of patients with potentially curable lesions. This usually requires that the tumor does not involve sites that would not be encompassed within the resection and that the tumor does not involve adjacent critical vascular structures such as the superior mesenteric artery (SMA) and vein (SMV), portal vein, celiac axis, or hepatic artery.

There are 2 approaches that might be taken to resolve this issue: a traditional approach and an alternative approach.

Traditional Approach

The traditional approach involves a contrast-enhanced helical CT scan with timed image sequences that permit evaluation of vascular structures and subtle metastatic implants (ie, CT angiography with phased images and thin cuts). The lack of major vascular involvement by tumor was associated with a resectability rate of more than 90%. Partial involvement of the SMV and/or SMA on CT angiography was associated with a resectability rate of 10% to 50% depending upon the extent of the vascular involvement.

Based upon this experience, our approach depends strongly upon the findings of CT angiography. For jaundiced patients with no involvement or minimal involvement of the major vessels and no evidence of distant metastases, we proceed directly to an attempt at surgical resection. For nonjaundiced patients (ie, those with body or tail tumors), or those with major but incomplete involvement of the vascular structures, we perform preoperative laparoscopy to exclude tiny metastases that might have been overlooked by CT. If the laparoscopy was negative, we then embark on a radical surgical resection. Finally, for those with circumferential involvement of one or more of the major vessels, we consider the lesion unresectable and proceed to obtain tissue for diagnosis and palliative nonoperative treatment.

Alternative Approach

Management of patients using the previously described traditional approach will result in operating on some 10% to 15% of patients with tumors that cannot be considered surgically "curable" (ie, they are found to invade the critical peripancreatic vascular structures, distant organs, or distant nodes at the time of attempted resection). Some have advocated performance of additional preoperative "staging" studies to identify such patients and spare them an unnecessary laparotomy. According to this alternative approach, patients with lesions felt to be potentially curable on the basis of helical CT angiography are studied further by magnetic resonance cholangiopancreatography (MRCP), EUS, laparoscopy, and/or laparoscopic US.

Diagnosing Pancreatic Cancer Algorithm

See Figure 32-3.

Staging of Pancreatic Exocrine Cancer

See Table 32-1.

In summary, CT is an appropriate initial imaging test because it detects tumors in the pancreas and can be used to stage for resectability and to detect liver metastases. The sensitivity of conventional CT for the diagnosis of tumors of less than 3 cm is 53% but the sensitivity of dual-phase spiral CT for resectable tumors is higher. However, the sensitivity of dual-phase spiral CT is related to the size of the tumor; the sensitivity for tumors of 0 to 15 mm is 67%, compared with 100% for tumors of greater than 15 mm.

EUS is the best test to detect small intrapancreatic tumors that cannot be detected by other imaging tests, and pancreatic cancers of 15 mm or less can be detected by EUS. EUS also may be used to obtain a tissue diagnosis at the time of the examination, particularly in patients with inconclusive CT results. Thus, EUS-guided fine needle aspiration is a safe and effective method to accurately diagnose and stage pancreatic cancer and possibly reduce cost by eliminating the need for additional tests or surgery.

Laparoscopy is used in some centers for staging because small hepatic and/or peritoneal metastases can be seen that are not visualized by less invasive tests. Although laparoscopy should not be done in all patients, it is indicated if there is a high likelihood of unresectability that has not been confirmed by imaging tests. Examples include pancreatic cancer and CT evidence of liver or other metastases that have not been proved with fine needle aspiration; pancreatic body or tail cancers, which have a very low chance of being resectable; and pancreatic cancer and ascites, which are probably caused by unrecognized peritoneal metastases.

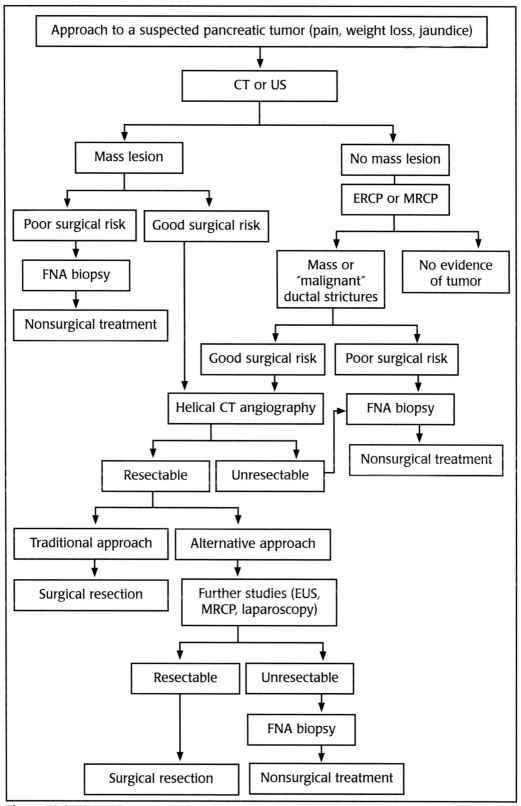

Figure 32-3. Diagnosing pancreatic cancer algorithm.

Table 32-1
Definition of TNM

Primary Tumor (T)

TX	Primary tumor cannot be assessed
T0	No evidence of primary tumor
Tis	In situ carcinoma
T1	Tumor limited to the pancreas, 2 cm or less in greatest dimension
T2	Tumor limited to the pancreas, more than 2 cm in greatest dimension
T3	Tumor extends beyond the pancreas but without involvement of the celiac axis or the superior mesenteric artery
T4	Tumor involves the celiac axis or the superior mesenteric artery (unresectable primary tumor)

Regional Lymph Nodes (N)

NX	Regional lymph nodes cannot be assessed
N0	No regional lymph node metastasis
N1	Regional lymph node metastasis

Distant Metastasis (M)

MX	Distant metastasis cannot be assessed
M0	No distant metastasis
M1	Distant metastasis

Stage Grouping

Stage 0	Tis, N0, M0
Stage IA	T1, N0, M0
Stage IB	T2, N0, M0
Stage IIA	T3, N0, M0
Stage IIB	T1-3, N1, M0
Stage III	T4, any N, M0
Stage IV	Any T, any N, M1

Bibliography

Conlon KC, Dougherty E, Klimstra DS, et al. The value of minimal access surgery in the staging of patients with potentially resectable peripancreatic malignancy. *Ann Surg.* 1996;223:134.

Conlon KC, Minnard EA. The value of laparoscopic staging in upper gastrointestinal malignancy. *Oncologist.* 1997;2:10.

Rosch T, Braig C, Gain T, et al. Staging of pancreatic and ampullary carcinoma by endoscopic ultrasonography. Comparison with conventional sonography, computed tomography and angiography. *Gastroenterology.* 1992;102:188.

Warshaw AL, Gu ZY, Wittenberg J, Waltman AC. Preoperative staging and assessment of resectability of pancreatic cancer. *Arch Surg.* 1990;125:230.

Wiersema MJ, Vilmann P, Giovanni M, et al. Endosongraphy-guided fine needle aspiration biopsy: diagnostic accuracy and complication assessment. *Gastroenterology.* 1997;112:1087.

WHAT ARE THE TREATMENT OPTIONS FOR EARLY AND LOCALLY ADVANCED PANCREATIC CANCER?

Paul S. Sepe, MD

Pancreatic cancer is the 4th leading cause of cancer death in the United States. In 2006, there were approximately 33,730 new cases with 32,300 deaths. Worldwide, incidence is approximately 217,000 new cases per year with 213,000 deaths. The lethality of pancreatic cancer stems largely from the fact that less than 20% of patients present with potentially resectable disease. While management of metastatic disease focuses mainly on palliation of symptoms and prolonging survival, the optimal therapy for early and locally advanced pancreatic cancer remains controversial and is currently the subject of intensive ongoing research.

Surgical management is the only curative option for patients with pancreatic cancer. However, cure rates for patients managed by surgery alone are extremely low, and as mentioned above, less than 20% of patients present with potentially resectable disease. Thus, researchers have focused on adjuvant chemotherapy and chemoradiotherapy in an effort to increase long-term survival. Traditionally, chemotherapeutic options have been largely centered around 5-fluorouracil (5-FU) containing regimens, although more recently, gemcitabine has been increasingly used. The majority of randomized control trials have been underpowered and provide conflicting results. Thus, significant controversy still exists regarding the optimal chemotherapeutic agent, appropriate dosing, the addition of concurrent radiotherapy, and the usefulness of neoadjuvant therapy.

Early pancreatic cancer is defined as stage I and II lesions that are amenable to surgical resection. The anatomic location of the tumor within the pancreas dictates the type of surgery performed. Lesions that are confined to the pancreatic head or uncinate process require pancreaticoduodenectomy (Whipple's procedure). Pylorus-preserving pancreaticoduodenectomy is also an option and seems to have comparable perioperative morbidity and mortality, without major differences in postoperative delayed gastric emptying or nutritional status. Surgeon preference and experience should dictate which operation to perform. Lesions that are located in the tail are removed with a distal pancreatectomy. Body lesions are approached according to their exact anatomic location. If they are closer to the pancreatic head, an extended pancreaticoduodenectomy may be performed. If closer to the tail, a distal subtotal pancreatectomy is performed.

Since greater than 50% of patients develop locoregional recurrence even after successful surgical resection with negative margins, adjuvant treatment with chemotherapy ± radiotherapy is currently recommended. The Gastrointestinal Tumor Study Group (GITSG) initially demonstrated a modest improvement in overall survival (20 months vs 11 months) when 5-FU chemotherapy was given with concurrent external beam radiotherapy (EBRT).[1] Unfortunately, the results of the European Organization for Research and Treatment of Cancer (EORTC) trial were unable to confirm a significant benefit for adjuvant chemoradiotherapy over resection alone.[2] In an attempt to answer the question regarding adjuvant therapy once and for all, the European Study Group for Pancreatic Cancer 1 trial (ESPAC-1) used a 2 X 2 factorial design assessing the benefit of adjuvant 5-FU chemotherapy alone, bolus 5-FU + radiotherapy, or chemoradiotherapy followed by additional chemotherapy, as compared to observation alone.[3] There was a significant survival benefit for adjuvant chemotherapy alone, but there was no significant benefit from radiotherapy. In fact, there was a trend toward worse survival for the group that received chemoradiotherapy. Unfortunately, the results of this trial were difficult to interpret due to high rate of protocol non-adherence and the lack of a separate analysis for each of the 4 groups in the 2 X 2 design.

More recently, the United States Intergroup has reported the results from a randomized phase III trial (RTOG-9704) that studied either postoperative infusional 5-FU followed by 5-FU + radiotherapy vs gemcitabine followed by 5-FU + radiotherapy.[4] There was significantly better overall survival in the gemcitabine arm for those patients with pancreatic head tumors (20.6 months vs 16.9 months). There was no significant difference for patients with pancreatic body/tail tumors. In addition, the CONKO-001 trial revealed a significant increase in disease-free survival for patients receiving gemcitabine adjuvant therapy vs observation alone (13.4 months vs 6.9 months).[5] Although survival was not a primary endpoint, there was a clear trend in favor of gemcitabine (22.1 months vs 20.2 months). However, this difference was not statistically significant (p=0.06).

There are theoretical benefits of preoperative neoadjuvant therapy, such as possible downstaging of the primary tumor and improvement of resection rate, as well as biologically staging patients so as to spare those who go on to develop metastatic disease the morbidity of surgery. Such therapy can be delivered safely without interfering with perioperative morbidity and mortality. However, there are no randomized control trials comparing neoadjuvant with adjuvant therapy.

Given the results of the above trials, current recommendations for the treatment of early pancreatic cancer differ between North America and Europe. The European approach emphasizes the results of EORTC and ESPAC-1 and does not include chemoradiation. The North American approach emphasizes the high risk of local failure and potential benefit of chemoradiotherapy. Thus, standard guidelines include radical pancreatic resection + postoperative 5-FU chemotherapy ± radiotherapy (Table 33-1). There is an emerging consensus that adjuvant chemotherapy with gemcitabine improves survival and represents an appropriate choice for current management and may be considered as a building block for future clinical trials.

Table 33-1

Treatment Options

Early Pancreatic Cancer	*Locally Advanced Pancreatic Cancer*
Radical pancreatic resection	Palliative surgical, percutaneous, and endoscopic procedures as appropriate
Postoperative 5-FU chemotherapy ± postoperative radiotherapy	External beam radiotherapy + 5-FU chemotherapy **OR** gemcitabine monotherapy

5-FU=5-fluorouracil.

Locally advanced pancreatic cancer refers to stage III disease with tumor extension to adjacent organs (lymph nodes, liver, duodenum, superior mesenteric artery, celiac trunk) such that complete surgical excision with negative pathologic margins is not possible. Depending on symptomatology and tumor location, these patients may benefit from palliation via endoscopic, surgical, or radiologic procedures. Biliary obstruction can be treated with stent placement by ERCP or percutaneous approaches. Gastric outlet obstruction can be managed by gastrojejunostomy or endoscopic placement of expandable metal stents. Chronic pain refractory to medication can be managed with celiac plexus neurolysis via percutaneous, radiologically guided or EUS-guided injection of steroids, analgesic agents, or ethanol.

Therapeutic options for locally advanced pancreatic cancer in the United States are mainly centered around chemoradiotherapy, although chemotherapy alone is becoming an increasingly utilized approach. Chemoradiotherapy has been mostly defined by 2 GITSG trials and an ECOG trial. The GITSG-9173 trial studied EBRT alone vs EBRT + bolus 5-FU.[6] The chemoradiation therapy arm was found to have significantly better 1-year survival (38% vs 11%). However, the E-8282 trial found no survival benefit when comparing EBRT to EBRT + infusional 5-FU + mitomycin.[7] Due to experience in other gastrointestinal malignancies, most notably rectal cancer, infusional 5-FU has largely supplanted bolus 5-FU as the most common approach. In this light, there is mounting evidence that oral capecitabine can safely replace infusional 5-FU as a radiation sensitizer. However, randomized control trials comparing these approaches are not available.

There have been few trials comparing chemoradiotherapy vs chemotherapy alone, and these have provided conflicting results. One notable study, a recent phase III study comparing 5-FU + cisplatin + EBRT initially followed by gemcitabine vs gemcitabine alone, found that gemcitabine monotherapy was less toxic and more effective (overall survival 13 months vs 8.6 months) than combination therapy.[8]

Studies looking at a stepwise approach of chemotherapy followed by chemoradiotherapy have supported this approach, but are comprised of only retrospective analysis. This offers the advantage of sparing those patients with rapidly progressive disease and subsequent metastasis from undergoing unnecessary radiotherapy.

Given the results of the above studies, optimal treatment for locally advanced pancreatic cancer remains controversial. Most would suggest external beam radiotherapy with concurrent low dose infusional 5-FU (see Table 33-1). Alternatively, gemcitabine mono-therapy may be used, but it should be recognized that there are no randomized control trials evaluating conventional EBRT + 5-FU vs gemcitabine monotherapy. Future clinical trials will need to be performed to further elucidate the optimal choice of chemoradio-therapy vs chemotherapy alone, as well as to explore novel therapeutic agents, such as paclitaxel, erlotinib, cetuximab, bevacizumab, and others.

References

1. Gastrointestinal Tumor Study Group. Further evidence of effective adjuvant combined radiation and chemo-therapy following curative resection of pancreatic cancer. *Cancer*. 1987;59:2006-2010.
2. Klinkenbijl JH, Jeekel J, Sahmoid T, et al. Adjuvant radiotherapy and 5-fluorouracil after curative resection of cancer of the pancreas and periampullary region: phase III trial of the EORTC gastrointestinal tract cancer cooperative group. *Ann Surg*. 1999;230:776-782.
3. Neoptolemos JP, Stocken DD, Friess H, et al. A randomized trial of chemoradiotherapy and chemotherapy after resection of pancreatic cancer. *N Engl J Med*. 2004;350:1200-1210.
4. Regine WF, Winter KA, Abrams RA, et al. Fluorouracil vs. gemcitabine chemotherapy before and after fluo-rouracil-based chemoradiation following resection of pancreatic adenocarcinoma: a randomized control trial. *JAMA*. 2008;299:1019-1026.
5. Oettle H, Post S, Neuhaus P, et al. Adjuvant chemotherapy with gemcitabine vs. observation in patients under-going curative-intent resection of pancreatic cancer: a randomized control trial. *JAMA*. 2007;297:267-277.
6. Gastrointestinal Tumor Study Group. A multi-institutional comparative trial of radiation therapy alone and in combination with 5-fluorouracil for locally unresectable pancreatic carcinoma. *Ann Surg*. 1979;189:205-208.
7. Cohen SJ, Dobelbower R, Lipsitz S, et al. A randomized phase III study of radiotherapy alone or with 5-fluorouracil and mitomycin-C in patients with locally advanced adenocarcinoma of the pancreas: Eastern Cooperative Oncology Group study E8282. *Int J Radiat Oncol Biol Phys*. 2005;62:1345-1350.
8. Chauffert B, Mornex F, Bonnetain F, et al. Phase III trial comparing intensive induction chemoradiotherapy (60 Gy, infusional 5-FU, and intermittent cisplatin) followed by maintenance gemcitabine with gemcitabine alone for locally advanced unresectable pancreatic cancer. Definitive results of the 2000-01 FFCD/SFRO study. *Ann Oncol*. 2008;19:1592-1599.

SECTION V

OTHER PANCREATIC NEOPLASMS

IN A PATIENT WITH RECURRENT HYPOGLYCEMIA, HOW DOES ONE EVALUATE FOR AN INSULINOMA?

Susan Ramdhaney, MD and Alphonso Brown, MD, MS Clin Epi

Endocrine tumors of the pancreas are extremely rare and comprise only 2% to 3% of all pancreatic tumors. Pancreatic endocrine tumors may be classified as secretory functioning tumors and nonsecretory indolent tumors. They can be single or multiple, benign or malignant. Insulinomas are the most common of the secreting pancreatic endocrine tumors and evolve from the cells of the ductular/acinar system. Insulinomas are usually solitary in nature and when present can occur anywhere within the pancreas. The multiple endocrine neoplasia syndrome type I is a rare condition in which multiple insulinomas may form.

Symptoms associated with insulinoma are secondary to the effects of insulin on the body. The most common symptoms associated with insulinomas include the neuroglycopenic symptoms such as dizziness, lethargy, amnesia, and confusion. Other symptoms that are sympathoadrenal include palpitations, diaphoresis, and tremulousness. Physicians should become suspicious in an individual with a pancreatic mass and symptoms of hypoglycemia.

The cardinal clinical feature of insulinoma is fasting hypoglycemia, which results from reduced hepatic glucose rather than increased glucose utilization. If an individual has a clinical suspicion of insulinoma, blood tests may be ordered to help assess the possibility of disease. Serum insulin levels and corresponding blood glucose levels are immediate tests. However, evaluation of true hypoglycemia via a 72-hour fast is necessary as part of the initial work-up. According to the Mayo Clinic protocol, blood specimens should be collected for measurement of plasma glucose, insulin, C-peptide, and proinsulin every 6 hours until the plasma glucose concentration is below 60 mg/dL (3.3 mmol/L) when these levels are monitored closely. The fast is ended when the plasma glucose concentration is 45 mg/dL (2.5 mmol/L) or less, the patient has symptoms or signs of hypoglycemia, 72

Figure 34-1. Linear array echo-endoscope for evaluation and biopsy of small pancreatic masses.

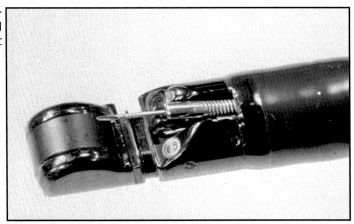

hours have elapsed, or when the plasma glucose concentration is less than 55 mg/dL (3 mmol/L) if Whipple's triad was documented on a prior occasion. When the fast is ended, plasma beta-hydroxybutyrate and sulfonylurea concentrations are measured, 1 mg of glucagon is given intravenously, and the plasma glucose measured 10, 20, and 30 minutes later or the patient is fed. Once these have been obtained, a determination of the ratio of serum insulin to blood glucose should be obtained. A ratio of 1 or greater is suggestive of insulinoma whereas a ratio of 0.4 or less suggests that an insulinoma is unlikely.

Once hypoglycemia is documented on a 72-hour fast, imaging studies are used to localize the tumor. Often insulinomas are smaller than 2 cm making the diagnosis extremely difficult. Currently imaging tests include spiral computed tomography (CT), arteriography, ultrasonography (transabdominal and endoscopic), 111In-pentetreotide imaging, and fluorine-18-L-dihydroxyphenylalanine positron emission tomography (18F-DOPA PET), with transabdominal ultrasound (US) being usually the first initial test used. In experienced hands, US will detect about 75% of insulinomas. In individuals with a negative US but in whom clinical suspicion of disease remains high, an endoscopic ultrasound (EUS), high-resolution CT, or a magnetic resonance imaging (MRI) study provides superior resolution and evaluation of the pancreas. These studies also have the advantage of being able to detect extremely small lesions. EUS evaluation also provides the added advantage of being able to biopsy any suspicious lesions (Figures 34-1 and 34-2).

If imaging and serum-based studies are still unable to reveal a lesion then other modalities, such as the use of hormones, may be used to diagnose insulinomas. Individuals who are given the pancreatic secretagogue secretin will not have the increase in serum insulin after being given secretin by vein. Somatostatin receptors are present on approximately 67% of insulinomas. Receptor scintigraphy using a radioisotope with antibodies that bind to somatostatin receptors can be used to identify insulinomas that have not been detected on imaging. Complex cases can be evaluated with the injection of calcium into the gastroduodenal, splenic, and superior mesenteric arteries with subsequent sampling of the hepatic venous effluent for insulin since calcium has been shown to stimulate insulin release in the area of the tumor.

Insulinomas tend to be slow growing and indolent lesions and early identification and removal of insulinomas are associated with excellent expected outcomes with low recurrence rates. However, if surgical resection is not possible, medical therapy such as

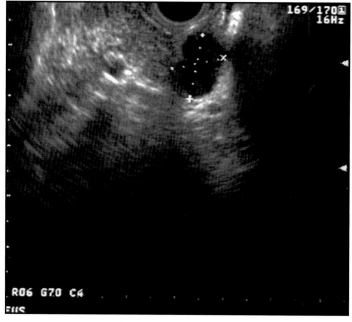

Figure 34-2. Endoscopic ultrasound images of small insulinoma in the body of the pancreas.

the use of diazoxide, which decreases insulin secretion, octreotide, which inhibits insulin secretion, and less effectively verapamil and phenytoin offer some benefit but none of these medical therapies are as effective as early detection and surgical resection. Options for hepatic resection of metastasis in certain cases include hepatic artery embolization, radiofrequency ablation, cryoablation, and liver transplantation. Recently, systemic chemotherapy with the use of streptozosin and doxorubicin had controversial results due to efficacy and toxicity issues, and novel approaches, such as the use of targeted radiotherapy, inhibitors of angiogenesis, and tyrosine kinase inhibitors, are being investigated.

Bibliography

Abboud B, Boujaoude J. Occult sporadic insulinoma: localization and surgical strategy. *World J Gastroenterol.* 2008;14(5):657-665.

Alexakis N, Neoptolemos JP. Pancreatic neuroendocrine tumours. *Best Pract Res Clin Gastroenterol.* 2008;22(1): 183-205.

Goldin SB, Aston J, Wahi MM. Sporadically occurring functional pancreatic endocrine tumors: review of recent literature. *Curr Opin Oncol.* 2008;20(1):25-33.

Tucker ON, Crotty PL, Conlon KC. The management of insulinoma. *Br J Surg.* 2006;93(3):264-275.

My Patient Has Chronic Diarrhea and Extensive Work-Up Has Been Negative. How to Establish a Diagnosis in a Patient Suspected of Having VIPoma?

Jack P. Braha, DO; Robin Baradarian, MD, FACG; and Nison Badalov, MD

Vasoactive intestinal peptide (VIP) is a peptide that inhibits gastric acid secretion in the stomach. In the small bowel, it stimulates chloride secretion and smooth muscle contraction. Other functions of VIP include serving as a neurotransmitter as well as modulator in potentiating the activity of acetylcholine in the salivary glands. As its name implies, VIP serves as a vasodilator elsewhere in the body including the coronary arteries. VIP acts on the myocardium as a positive inotrope and chronotrope. During its circulation throughout the bloodstream, VIP has a half-life of approximately 2 minutes.

Vasoactive intestinal peptide tumors (VIPoma) fall into the category of non-α, non-β islet-cell pancreatic endocrine tumors. Other pancreatic endocrine tumors include gastrinoma, insulinoma, glucagonoma, somatostatinoma, GRFoma, ACTHoma, carcinoid syndrome, parathyroid-related protein tumors, and nonfunctional tumors. Pancreatic endocrine tumors occur in 0.5% to 1.5% of autopsies but are only clinically apparent in 1:100,000 of the population. These tumors make up only a small number, 1% to 2%, of detected pancreatic neoplasms.

Patients with vasoactive intestinal peptide tumors often present with a syndrome of symptoms known as WDHA (watery diarrhea, hypokalemia, and achlorhydria). Clinical manifestations of VIPoma are often episodic, dispersed between symptom-free periods. The secretory nature of diarrhea that is found in patients with VIPomas is secondary to

Figure 35-1. Endoscopic ultrasound image of the body of the pancreas showing an 8-mm vasoactive intestinal polypeptide-secreting tumor in the head of the pancreas not identified on computed tomography and magnetic resonance imaging.

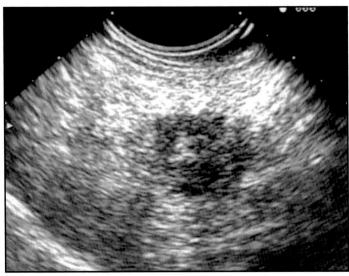

the peptide's action upon chloride (Cl-) channels. After activating adenylyl cyclase receptors on secretory cells located within the intestinal crypts, cAMP is generated and opens apical Cl- channels. Once the secretion of Cl- begins, water and sodium are soon to follow. A secretory diarrhea, also known as "pancreatic cholera," then follows, similar to that associated with bacterial toxins from Vibrio cholera and enterotoxigenic E. coli.

Patients with VIPoma have voluminous diarrhea, often in excess of 3 to 5 L/day. Given its secretory nature, this does not respond to fasting. The excessive secretory state leads to dehydration, hypokalemia, hypercalcemia, hyperglycemia, and extraintestinal manifestations such as flushing, palpitations, fatigue, and weakness. VIP hypersecretion also amplifies its inhibitory effects on the secretion of gastric acid leading to hypo- or achlorhydria with hypochloremic metabolic alkalosis.

Once a clinician obtains a history suggestive of VIPoma, it is imperative to obtain a fasting plasma VIP level. Given the episodic nature of symptoms in VIPoma patients, multiple VIP levels should be measured to ensure that a VIPoma is not missed during a clinically silent period. Next, imaging to locate the suspect tumor should be obtained. Generally, computed tomography scan with intravenous contrast locates most VIPomas. The most sensitive imaging modality, endoscopic ultrasound, is invasive but can be used to better identify suspect lesions, especially those less than 1 cm, and offers the ability to obtain fine needle aspiration at the same time (Figure 35-1). EUS with fine needle aspiration offers a diagnostic accuracy of 80% for pancreatic adenocarcinoma but only 46% for pancreatic endocrine tumors. Other imaging modalities include somatostatin receptor scintigraphy, magnetic resonance imaging and angiography. In patients with symptoms consistent with VIPoma and an elevated plasma VIP level (>500 pg/mL) but lacking conclusive imaging, VIPoma should still be suspected.

Management of VIPoma can be achieved by either medical or surgical therapy. Initial medical therapy should be focused on fluid resuscitation in the dehydrated patient and maintenance of electrolyte balance. Symptomatic therapy is often effective with administration somatostatin. This leads to inhibitory effects on secretory and motor functions that are affected by the VIP hypersecretion. Although somatostatin has a 2-minute half-life in the serum, similar to VIP, the synthetic analogue octreotide with a half-life of over 1 hour is available for subcutaneous administration. Sandostatin LAR Depot (Novartis, Basel, Switzerland) is a once-monthly depot injection of octreotide that can be substituted for better patient adherence and convenience. While octreotide is successful in reducing symptoms in the majority of patients, tachyphylaxis develops within 1 year of treatment and titration is required to keep symptoms controlled. In refractory cases, the addition of glucocorticoids has been successful in controlling symptoms.

Currently, surgical resection is the only curative modality and the treatment of choice for locoregional pancreatic endocrine tumors, including VIPoma. Eligible candidates should be referred to specialty centers for pancreatic surgery. Surgery is also considered for patients with metastatic disease to the liver if the hepatic mass is amenable to resection. The same applies for metastatic lung lesions that can be resected for cure. Patients with metastatic disease not amenable to surgical cure, depending on location of the tumor, may undergo chemotherapy, radiofrequency ablation, or radiotherapy. Successful chemotherapeutic agents include doxorubicin/streptozocin, dacarbazine, capecitabine, 5-fluorouracil, temozolomide, and interferon. Treatment with synthetic somatostatin should be provided to all symptomatic patients.

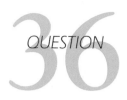
MY PATIENT HAS REFLUX ESOPHAGITIS IN SPITE OF DAILY OMEPRAZOLE. HIS SERUM GASTRIN ON OMEPRAZOLE IS 750. WHAT IS THE NEXT STEP IN EVALUATION FOR GASTRINOMA?

Susan Truong, HMS III and Alphonso Brown, MD, MS Clin Epi

Reflux esophagitis is best treated with anti-secretory therapy, proton pump inhibitors (PPIs). The step-up approach for heartburn, reflux esophagitis, beginning with over-the-counter antacids, progressing to H2 blockers, and then PPIs, has been replaced with a step-down approach. As the cost of PPIs, with the advent of generic omeprazole, has decreased, this approach is not effective and not cost effective. PPIs are considered just as safe as H2 blockers, yet they are far more effective.

Years prior, when PPIs were first introduced as omeprazole (Prilosec [AstraZeneca, Wilmington, DE]), safety was a concern. As omeprazole resulted in a profound decrease in acid secretion, the cells responsible for stimulating acid secretion, sensing the absence of acid, increased release of the stimulatory hormone, gastrin. Although gastrin levels normally rise in patients taking PPIs, the elevation is typically not of clinical significance. Animal studies, especially murine models, given PPIs have shown a proliferation of gastrin-secreting cells and even the development of gastrinomas. The fear has been that the elevated gastrin level (hypergastrinemia) often seen in patients on PPIs will pose a risk for persons to develop gastrinomas.

Hypergastrinemia can be caused by several entities (Table 36-1) with gastrinoma, or Zollinger-Ellison syndrome (ZES), the most feared the diagnosis. A normal fasting serum gastrin level typically is below 110 to 150 pg/mL. Antisecretory medications can moderately raise the gastrin level to approximately 200 to 400 pg/mL. It has been shown, howev-

Table 36-1

Causes of Hypergastrinemia

Cause	Gastrin Level (pg/mL)	Comments
Elevated antral pH		
Truncal vagotomy without antrectomy	~200	Post surgical
H2 receptor antagonist therapy	~200	
Proton pump inhibitor therapy	~200 to 400	
Chronic atrophic gastritis from H. pylori	~200 to 400	pH >4.0
Chronic atrophic gastritis from pernicious anemia	>1000	pH >4.0
Gastrin-secreting tumors		Secretin stimulation:
Gastrinoma	>1000	dramatic rise in gastrin levels

Adapted from Orlando LA, Lenard L, Orlando RC. Chronic hypergastrinemia: causes and consequences. *Dig Dis Sci.* 2007;52:2482-2489.

er, that a group of approximately 5% of patients on PPI therapy have gastrin levels greater than 400 pg/mL. With gastrinomas, one typically sees fasting gastrin levels greater than 1000 pg/mL but it is important to remember that as many as 10% of ZES patients have serum gastrins well below 1000 pg/mL.

ZES typically presents with recurrent multiple peptic ulcer disease due to acid hypersecretion. Approximately 90% of patients develop multiple ulcers with the majority located in the first portion of the duodenum. ZES can also present with diarrhea as the predominant symptom as excess acid secretion can lead to inactivation of pancreatic enzymes resulting in malabsorption and steatorrhea. Signs suggestive of acid hypersecretion, such as multiple recurrent peptic ulcer disease, diarrhea, or history of multiple endocrine neoplasia type I, should prompt work-up for ZES. This includes fasting serum gastrin concentration off of PPIs, secretin stimulation test, and gastric acid secretion studies. The first 2 tests are routinely used to aid in diagnosis.

The first step is to obtain a fasting gastrin level off of PPI therapy for at least 1 week. As mentioned above, a gastrin greater than 1000 pg/mL is typically seen in ZES. It is, however, not diagnostic of the disease as patients with pernicious anemia can also have serum gastrin levels in that range. It is, therefore, important to keep the patient's clinical picture in mind when evaluating for gastrinoma. For patients with serum gastrins greater than 1000 pg/mL, a gastric pH probe can help to distinguish between chronic atrophic gastritis and other causes. An elevated pH would suggest pernicious anemia. For patients with gastrin levels between 110 pg/mL and 1000 pg/mL, a secretin stimulation test can help guide further work-up. This test is based on the fact that a normal gastrin-secreting cell will be inhibited by the infusion of secretin (a normally acting inhibitor of gastrin secretion). Patients with ZES, with a gastrinoma, have an uncoupling of the secretin inhibitory receptor. Thus, these patients should have a persistent or significant elevation of serum gastrin levels after secretin stimulation while patients with other causes for

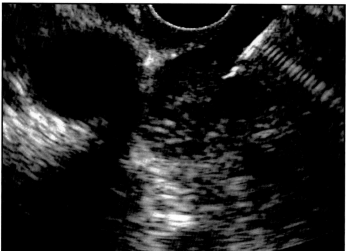

Figure 36-1. Endoscopic ultrasound showing a small 1.5-cm mass consistent with an islet cell tumor. Fine needle aspiration shown revealed gastrin-secreting cells on immunostain consistent with gastrinoma.

hypergastrinemia should not have a rise in serum gastrin. A decrease should be noted. If a patient has no inhibitory response to the secretin, one should pursue imaging to try to localize the tumor. This can be done either with an octreotide scan or an endoscopic ultrasound (EUS). Octreoscan is best for metastatic disease or lymph node involvement. EUS images the pancreas with great accuracy and can allow a fine needle aspiration of small suspected tumors to confirm the diagnosis (Figure 36-1).

For this particular patient, an elevated serum gastrin of 750 pg/mL on PPI therapy is not strong enough evidence to suggest gastrinoma. Several options exist, including a secretin stimulation test. With ZES being such a rare entity, one should consider all other causes for his PPI resistant reflux esophagitis before pursuing this pathway. The first reasonable step would be for the patient to have endoscopy to evaluate his reflux and to determine if he has gastritis or ulcer disease as well. Should this reveal multiple duodenal ulcers, one may pursue a repeat gastrin level after stopping PPI for 1 week. Computed tomography, magnetic resonance imaging, and EUS should be performed for imaging if a gastrinoma is suspected.

Bibliography

Koop HAR. Long-term maintenance treatment of reflux esophagitis with omeprazole: prospective study in patients with H2-blocker-resistant esophagitis. *Dig Dis Sci.* 1991;36;552-557.

Lamberts R, Brunner G, Solcia E. Effects of very long (up to 10 years) proton pump blockade on human gastric mucosa. *Digestion.* 2001;64:205-213.

Orlando LA, Lenard L, Orlando RC. Chronic hypergastrinemia: causes and consequences. *Dig Dis Sci.* 2007;52:2482-2489.

Warner RR. Enteroendocrine tumors other than carcinoid: a review of clinically significant advances. *Gastroenterology.* 2005;128:1668-1684.

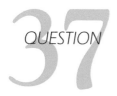
WHAT MASSES MIMIC PANCREATIC CANCER?

Susan Truong, HMS III and Alphonso Brown, MD, MS Clin Epi

More frequently, pancreatic masses are discovered incidentally during diagnostic imaging (Table 37-1). Pancreatic ductal adenocarcinoma is the most common tumor mass of the pancreas, accounting for more than 80% of all pancreatic tumors and an additional 10% of pancreatic tumors are atypical variants of ductal adenocarcinoma. While the classic pancreatic ductal adenocarcinoma has a very characteristic appearance on diagnostic imaging, the remaining variants may be difficult to distinguish. This poses a difficult problem for diagnosis and clinical management. Tuberculosis and fungal and parasitic infections can result from hematogenous spread or infiltration from peripancreatic lymph nodes. Tuberculosis in the pancreas may appear as a single focal lesion mimicking pancreatic adenocarcinoma (Figure 37-1).

A variety of inflammatory pseudotumoral lesions often are mistaken for pancreatic cancer on imaging. One such entity is pseudotumorous pancreatitis. This focal, noncalcified mass occasionally results from chronic pancreatitis and can have the radiological appearance of pancreatic cancer (Figure 37-2). In one study, 21 patients who were radiologically considered to have carcinoma or islet cell tumors were found at histological diagnosis to have chronic relapsing pancreatitis. Infectious masses can also appear as tumor-like lesions on imaging. An exceedingly rare cause of pancreatic mass is intrapancreatic splenosis. This ectopic splenic tissue can be very difficult to distinguish from a pancreatic cancer. Other solid lesions that can mimic pancreatic cancer include lymphoma and metastatic disease. Solid masses should be evaluated for resectability. When there is diagnostic doubt, an endoscopic ultrasound (EUS) with fine needle aspiration may be considered for further work-up.

Cystic pancreatic lesions are the minority of pancreatic masses. They can have one of three broad etiologies: congenital, inflammatory, and neoplastic. Of the non-neoplastic

Table 37-1

Classification of Masses in the Pancreas

Pancreatic Masses	*Cystic*	*Solid*
Non-neoplastic	I. Congenital: true cysts, choledochocele, syndromes associated with cysts (von Hippel-Lindau, cystic fibrosis) II. Inflammatory: pseudocysts, abscess, hydatid cyst	I. Inflammatory: pseudotumorous pancreatitis, infectious tumor-like masses (tuberculosis, fungal, parasitic infections) II. Other: ectopic spleen (splenosis) III. Autoimmune
Neoplastic	I. Benign: serous cystadenoma, cystic teratoma II. Malignant (or potentially malignant): mucinous cystic neoplasm, solid and papillary epithelial neoplasm (solid-pseudopapillary tumor), intraductal papillary mucinous neoplasm, cystic islet cell tumors, acinar cell cystic tumors	I. Exocrine: PanIN, pancreatic-infiltrating ductal adenocarcinoma, anaplastic carcinoma, adenosquamous carcinoma, mucinous noncystic carcinoma, pancreatoblastoma, undifferentiated carcinoma with osteoclast-like giant cells II. Endocrine: islet cell tumors (insulinoma, gastrinoma, VIPoma, glucagonoma, somatostatinoma, pancreatic carcinoid) III. Other: metastatic disease, lymphoma, sarcoma, paraganglioma

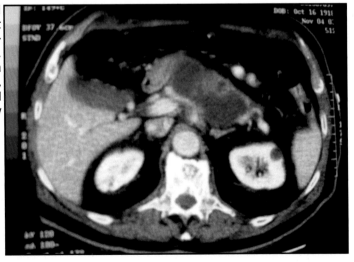

Figure 37-1. This mass found on computed tomographic scan was performed on a 45-year-old Nigerian physician. Despite appearing to be a stage II pancreatic carcinoma, biopsy of the mass revealed acid fast bacilli, cultures grew mycobacterium tuberculosis.

pancreatic cysts, pseudocysts are by far the most common accounting for approximately 90% of all cystic lesions. They are localized collections of necrotic/hemorrhagic material and can be found within the pancreatic parenchyma or more commonly, adjacent to it in the peripancreatic tissues. Intrapancreatic pseudocysts may even communicate with the ductal system. Pancreatic pseudocysts generally result from the intense inflammatory

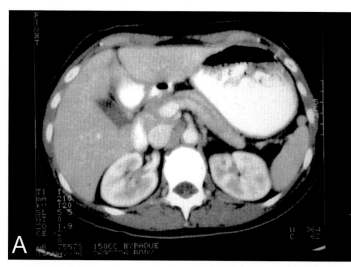

Figure 37-2. (A) This 38-year-old woman had epigastric pain, nausea, and weight loss. Computed tomography revealed a mass in the head of her pancreas with proximal ductal dilatation. (B) After resection of the head of the pancreas (Frey procedure), histology showed diffuse fibrosis. Genetic analysis confirmed the diagnosis of cationic trypsinogen mutation–hereditary pancreatitis.

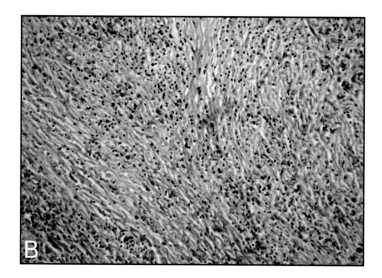

response and autodigestion associated with acute pancreatitis. Computed tomography (CT) and EUS are usually effective in diagnosing pancreatic pseudocysts, but if there is doubt, CT- or US-guided fine needle aspiration will secure the diagnosis. Other inflammatory cystic lesions include abscess and ecchinococcal (hydatid) cysts.

Congenital cysts are believed to result from abnormal development of the pancreatic ducts and range in size from microscopic to up to 5 cm in diameter. They can be associated with certain hereditary disorders such as polycystic diseases, cystic fibrosis, and von Hippel-Lindau syndrome. Patients with von Hippel-Lindau syndrome generally have retinal and central nervous system vascular neoplasms as well as congenital cysts of the pancreas, liver, and kidney. A choledochocele, or congenital bile duct cyst, may also present as a cystic mass near the pancreas.

Neoplastic cysts range in their malignant potential. Serous cystadenomas and cystic teratomas are almost always benign. Conversely, mucinous cystadenomas have the potential to develop into malignant mucinous cystadenocarcinoma. Since there is considerable

Figure 37-3. A 55-year-old man presented with elevated bilirubin and weight loss. Endoscopic ultrasound of the pancreas revealed a hypoechoic mass in the head of the pancreas. There was no history of alcoholism. Computed tomography, magnetic resonance imaging, and transabdominal ultrasound were all normal. Only a fullness to the head of the pancreas with a mass effect was seen. Serum immunoglobulin G4 was profoundly elevated. Suspecting autoimmune pancreatitis, prednisone was given. Laboratory and imaging abnormalities resolved over 2 weeks.

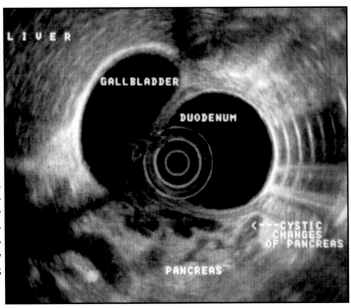

overlap in the appearance of these lesions on initial CT imaging, further diagnostic work-up is generally warranted, which includes magnetic resonance cholangiopancreatography, EUS with fine needle aspiration, and biochemical testing.

Autoimmune pancreatitis (Figure 37-3) can also present as a mass in the pancreas. The middle-aged patient with a mass in the pancreas, double duct sign, and elevated bilirubin is suspected as having pancreatic cancer. In recent years, it has become more apparent that a small number of these patients with classical signs of pancreatic cancers have autoimmune pancreatitis. This disorder responds well to steroids and is discussed elsewhere.

In summary, although pancreatic cancer is common, it is important to establish the diagnosis by biopsy. All pancreatologists describe cases of patients who either underwent unnecessary surgery or were left to die of pancreatic cancer only to have been found to have another diagnosis. It is important for clinicians to address the possibility of benign cystic disease, infectious diseases, and chronic inflammatory conditions, including autoimmune pancreatitis.

Bibliography

Degan L, Wiesner W, Beglinger C. Cystic and solid lesions of the pancreas. *Best Pract Res Clin Gastroenterol.* 2008;22(1):91-103.

De Juan C, Sanchez M, Miquel R, Pages M, Ayuso JR, Ayuso C. Uncommon tumors and pseudotumoral lesions of the pancreas. *Curr Probl Diagn Radiol.* 2008;37:145-164.

Lammer J, Herlinger H, Zalaudek G, Hofler H. Pseudotumorous pancreatitis. *Gastrointest Radiol.* 1985;10(1):59-67.

Rafique A, Freeman S, Carroll N. A clinical algorithm for the assessment of pancreatic lesions: utilization of 16- and 64- section multidetector CT and endoscopic ultrasound. *Clin Radiol.* 2007;62:1142-1153.

Sica GT, Reed MF. Intrapancreatic accessory spleen. *Radiology.* 2000;217:134-137.

SECTION VI

BILIARY

WHAT IS THE ROLE OF CHOLANGIOPANCREATOSCOPY IN PANCREATICOBILIARY DISEASE?

Greg Guthrie, MD, and Young Lee, MD

Cholangioscopy refers to the insertion of an endoscope into the biliary system with subsequent direct visualization of the bile ducts. It has existed for many years and in many different forms—percutaneously by radiologists, intraoperatively by surgeons, and endoscopically as an extension of endoscopic retrograde cholangiopancreatography (ERCP). This later endoscopic form is often referred to as "peroral" approach and is accomplished via retrograde insertion of miniature endoscopes through the ampulla of Vater. The peroral approach will be the main focus of the remainder of this chapter (Figures 38-1 and 38-2).

The ability to directly visualize biliary pathology provides a significant advantage over conventional ERCP in multiple disease states. This includes the evaluation of biliary strictures, the evaluation of large or atypical filling defects within the common bile duct (CBD), and more definitive therapy for resistant CBD stones. As technology advances, the indications should continue to expand.

There are several different cholangioscopes commercially available in the United States and they are listed in Table 38-1. These endoscopes fit through the channel of a typical therapeutic duodenoscope (42 mm) and can be inserted via wire-guidance using a 0.035-inch or 0.025-inch wire under fluoroscopy. In addition to the endoscope, other accessories are often required including cytology brushes, biopsy forceps, and electrohydraulic lithotripsy (EHL) probes.

There are pitfalls in performing cholangioscopy that limit its use and availability. The first major limitation is handling and using a dual endoscope system. Some endoscope systems are very large and bulky and necessitate 2 separate endoscopists—one to operate the "mother" duodenoscope and one to operate the "baby" cholangioscope. The next limitation has to do with the endoscopes themselves. These scopes can have limited

Figure 38-1. Fluoroscopic image of pancreatoscopy with Spy Glass (Boston Scientific Corp, Marlboro, MA).

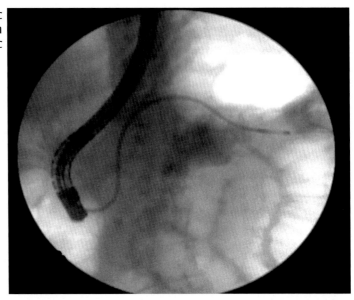

Figure 38-2. Endoscopic view of the pancreatic duct from Spy Glass (Boston Scientific Corp, Marlboro, MA) showing early adenocarcinoma. Direct endoscopic biopsy confirmed diagnosis.

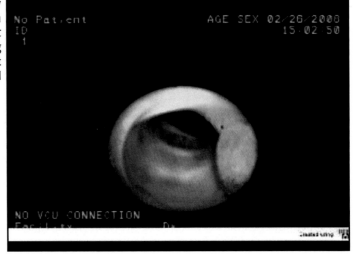

Table 38-1

Commercially Available Cholangioscopes

	Olympus	*Pentax*	*Pentax*	*Boston Scientific*
Model	CHF BP 30	FCP-9N	FCP-8P	Spy Glass
Working channel	1.2 mm	1.2 mm	0.75 mm	1.2 mm
Diameter	3.4 mm	3.1 mm	2.8 mm	3.33 mm

maneuverability with only 2-way tip deflection, significant fragility making them easily damaged by the elevator of the duodenoscope, and less-than-ideal endoscopic views in some systems. Finally, due to size most cholangioscopes do not fit through a normal caliber papilla necessitating sphincterotomy in almost all patients with all the inherent risks that go with this.

Current data suggest there is an advantage over cholangiography. One study in 97 patients with bile duct strictures found cholangiography with a combination of cytology and blind biopsies correctly identified 22 of 38 malignant strictures and 35 of 38 benign strictures. According to Tischendorf et al,[1] the addition of cholangioscopy increased the diagnostic yield to 38 of 38 malignant lesions and 33 of 35 benign lesions. In addition, cholangioscopy also has shown significant benefit it patients with primary sclerosing cholangitis (PSC). In 53 patients with PSC and dominant strictures, ERCP with brushings was compared to cholangioscopy with biopsy. According to Arya et al,[2] cholangioscopy was superior in its sensitivity (92% vs 66%), specificity (93% vs 51%), and accuracy (93% vs 55%).

Cholangioscopy for fragmentation of large or recalcitrant stones is a major indication. To accomplish this, EHL probes are placed through the cholangioscope and then used to fragment the stones under direct visualization with high power shock waves. Results published by Wiedmann et al[3] have shown a very high success rate (90% to 100%) in achieving complete CBD clearance. In addition, it may decrease the number of endoscopic sessions needed to obtain complete CBD clearance.

The technology of this modality continues to improve. Smaller, more maneuverable cholangioscopes with a better resolution continue to be developed. In addition, other cholangioscopic modalities are becoming available including multiband imaging via cholangioscopes and photodynamic therapy via cholangioscopy for cholangiocarcinoma.

Pancreatoscopy is an evolving complementary test to other imaging modalities available in evaluating pancreatic diseases. During ERCP, the pancreatic duct is cannulated with a conventional cannulatome. Subsequently, a cannulatome is exchanged for a pancreatoscope which is advanced through the biopsy channel of therapeutic duodenoscope into the pancreatic orifice allowing direct luminal imaging of the pancreatic duct. As a result, image-guided forcep biopsies, use of baskets, placement of stents, dilatation of strictures, and endotherapy for stones can be applied. Secretin 100 U intravenously can be given to stimulate the exocrine function of the pancreas and make the visual field clear.

Cholangiopancreatoscopes

An intact pancreatic sphincter and a small size as well as the tortuosity of the pancreatic duct are significant anatomic hurdles. Currently available pancreatoscopes are often too large to cannulate a normal caliber pancreatic duct and the smaller ultrathin pancreatoscope is limited by fragility, lack of maneuverability, absence of irrigation, no accessory channel, and poor imaging resolution. Additionally, pancreatic anatomical anomalies such as pancreas divisum, annular pancreas, and surgically altered anatomy may be difficult to access through currently available pancreatoscopes. With improvements of pancreatoscopes, currently available endoscopic imaging technology may be able to be incorporated such as narrow band imaging, multiband imaging, I-Scan, high definition, and finally confocal microscopy.

Table 38-2
Pancreatoscopy Findings in Normal and Diseased States of the Pancreas

Pathology	*Pancreatoscopy Findings*
Normal pancreas	Smooth whitish-pink mucosa, distinct capillary appearance
Chronic pancreatitis	Protein plugs, calcified stones, rough whitish mucosa, scar formation, edema, erythema, indistinct capillary appearance
Pancreatic cancer	Stenoses or duct cut-off, friable mucosa with erosion, compression
Intraductal papillary mucinous tumors	Papillary tumors, oval shaped, nodular/villous, whitish, spotty or linear redness

Pancreatitis appears to complicate about 1.8% of patients undergoing pancreatoscopy especially when sphincterotomy and sphincter dilatation are utilized to access the duct. Risks such as bleeding, infection, and perforation inherent to ERCP are also present. Seeding of cancer along the duct is a potential consideration. Finally, ductal disruption and iatrogenic ductal injury are of concern secondary to instrument trauma.

The current role of pancreatoscopy is still evolving. It plays a significant role in evaluating intraductal papillary mucinous tumors (IPMT), a slow-growing pancreatic ductal epithelial tumor (Table 38-2). Not only can it help distinguish benign from malignant IPMT by allowing targeted forcep biopsy but it allows more accurate preoperative mapping of involved portions of the pancreas prior to surgical resection. Pancreatoscopy also plays a role in chronic pancreatitis both in the evaluation of equivocal strictures and the treatment of intraductal stones that failed traditional extraction methods. Screening ductal evaluation of patients who are high risk for pancreatic cancer, such as those with strong family history, history of recurrent pancreatitis, and those with late onset diabetes mellitus, appears to be promising. Endoscopic evaluation of peripancreatic fluid collection such as pseudocyst through the disrupted duct has also been reported. For now, this exciting new technology should be used on highly selected patients with an individualized approach to patient care. How the findings will affect the management of a particular patient with pancreaticobiliary disease must be addressed prior to the intervention.

References

1. Tischendorf JJ, Kruger M, Trautwein C, et al. Cholangioscopic characterization of dominant bile duct stenoses in patients with primary sclerosing cholangitis. *Endoscopy.* 2006;38:665-669.
2. Arya N, Nelles SE, Haber GB, Kim YI, Kortan PK. Electrohydraulic lithotripsy in 111 patients: a safe and effective therapy for difficult bile duct stones. *Am J Gastroenterol.* 2004;99:2330-2334.
3. Wiedmann MW, Caca K. General principles of photodynamic therapy (PDT) and gastrointestinal applications. *Curr Pharm Biotechnol.* 2004;5:397-408.

Bibliography

Arisaka Y, Masuda D, Kawakami K, Miyaji K, Katsu K-I. Peroral pancreatoscopy: current status and future expectations using narrow band imaging. *Digestive Endoscopy.* 2007;19(Suppl 1):S79-S86.

ASGE practice guideline. Cholangiopancreatoscopy. *Gastrointest Endosc.* 2008;68(3):411-421.

Fukuda Y, Tsuyuguchi T, Sakai Y, Tsuchiya S, Saisyo H. Diagnostic utility of peroral cholangioscopy for various bile-duct lesions. *Gastrointest Endosc.* 2005;62(3):374-382.

Kelsy PB. Cholangioscopy. In: Baron TH, Kozarek R, Carr-Locke DL, eds. *ERCP.* Philadelphia, PA: Saunders; 2008: 211-217.

Kodama T, Koshitani T, Sato H. Electronic pancreatoscopy for the diagnosis of pancreatic diseases. *Am J Gastroenterol.* 2002;97:617-622.

Kodama T, Sato H, Horii Y. Pancreatoscopy for the next generation: development of the peroral electronic pancreatoscope system. *Gastrointest Endosc.* 1999;49:366-371.

Yamao K, Ohashi K, Nakamura T, et al. Efficacy of peroral pancreatoscopy in the diagnosis of pancreatic diseases. *Gastrointest Endosc.* 2003;57(2):205-209.

Yasuda K, Sakata M, Ueda M, Uno K, Nakajima M. The use of pancreatoscopy in the diagnosis of intraductal papillary mucinous tumor lesions of the pancreas. *Clinical Gastroenterology and Hepatology.* 2005;3(7 Suppl 1): S53-S57.

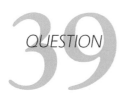
MY PATIENT HAD A MAGNETIC RESONANCE CHOLANGIOPANCREATOGRAPHY TO EVALUATE FOR COMMON BILE DUCT STONES, BUT THE READING INCLUDES A "DOUBLE DUCT SIGN." WHAT DOES THIS MEAN? DOES IT NEED ENDOSCOPIC RETROGRADE CHOLANGIOPANCREATOGRAPHY?

Hui Hing (Jack) Tin, MD and Jai Mirchandani, MD

Although controversial in the past, the current accepted term, *double duct sign*, refers to narrowing of both the pancreatic and the common bile duct with dilatation of the ducts proximal to the site of narrowing. It is usually discovered through such studies such as magnetic resonance cholangiopancreatography (MRCP) (Figures 39-1 and 39-2), endoscopic retrograde cholangiopancreatography (ERCP), computed tomography (CT) scan (Figure 39-3), and transabdominal or endoscopic ultrasounds (EUS). These studies are usually prompted by obstructive jaundice and other signs and symptoms including abdominal pain, anorexia, abnormal liver function tests, weight lost, cholelithiasis, and choledocholithiasis.

Figure 39-1. Magnetic resonance cholangiopancreatography showing double duct sign: dilatation of both the common bile duct and pancreatic duct from either strictures or external compression.

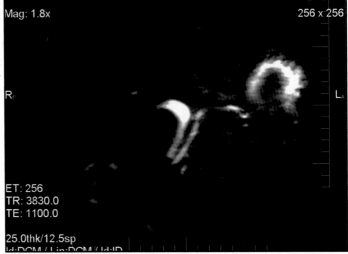

Figure 39-2. Full-size magnetic resonance cholangiopancreatography of the patient from Figure 39-1.

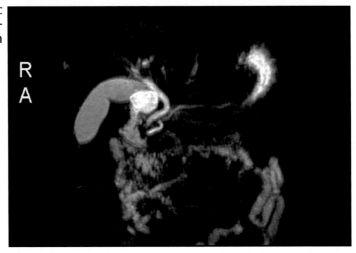

The significance of double duct sign is its high predictive value for pancreatiobiliary malignancy. In a study by Kalady et al[1] of 355 patients, the double duct sign was found to have a sensitivity of 77%, positive predictive value of 65%, specificity of 79.9%, and a negative predictive value of 87.6%. In one Japanese study,[2] its positive predictive value can be as high as 80%. Combined with other ductal characteristics, such as severe stenosis and marked proximal dilatations, it is a very useful indicator of malignancies. Benign causes of the double duct sign include chronic pancreatitis, pancreatic pseudocyst, pancreatic duct stones, pancreas divisum, and, in one case report, *Strongyloides Stercoralis* infection.

The formation of the double duct sign is postulated as a mass at the head of the pancreas or at the ampulla compressing both the distal ends of the common bile duct and pancreatic duct causing an obstruction and dilatation of the ducts. In cases where there is no obvious mass, stricture formation from ductal pancreatic carcinoma or cholangiocarcinoma is felt to be the culprit. In chronic pancreatitis, scar tissue formation in the pancreas causes strictures and dilatation of the ducts. Many studies have been done to look at the size, length, irregularity, and location of the strictures to better differentiate malignant and benign strictures radiologically, although the results are currently inconclusive.[3]

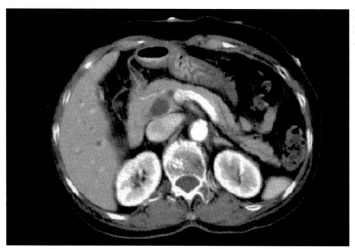

Figure 39-3. Computed tomography scan of patient with double duct sign.

In general, EUS, helical CT scan, and MRCP/magnetic resonance imaging (MRI) are accurate means for the detection of pancreatic adenocarcinoma and determination of resectability. If the patient is deemed a surgical candidate, ERCP would not be needed. Preoperative ERCP does not add further staging information and may result in complications (pancreatitis, perforation) that may make operative intervention more difficult and/or may considerably delay operative intervention resulting in a decreased potential for curative resection. If an MRCP/MRI or helical CT scan does not reveal an obvious mass or cyst at the head of the pancreas, rather than starting the work-up with ERCP, a less invasive option would be to pursue further evaluation with an EUS with biopsy and fine needle aspiration if a mass can be visualized. This is also a less invasive way to evaluate the ampulla as well.

ERCP serves 2 purposes in a patient with the double duct sign. If no obvious mass is seen on the radiologic study such as MRI or CT scan, the ERCP can be of value. It can serve as a diagnostic tool for tissue confirmation via forceps biopsy, needle aspiration, bile or pancreatic juice aspiration, and brush biopsy for ductal pancreatic carcinoma, however, as noted above this should not be first line.[4] ERCP can also be used for confirmation of the diagnosis to guide chemotherapeutic treatment in patients who are not surgical candidates secondary to unresectability and/or co-morbid medical conditions. The sensitivity rate for ERCP-directed brush cytology or biopsy is 30% to 50%, with a combination achieving sensitivity rates of 65% to 70%.[5] Techniques to enhance the accuracy of cytology and pancreatic juice appear to be significant, but are experimental or not widely available. The second and most important purpose of ERCP is it can be used for palliation with insertion of metallic or plastic stents for relief of obstructive symptoms from the strictures. In general, the self-expanding metal stents (SEMS) are preferred over the plastic stents if the patient's life expectancy is greater than 4 months. This is because plastic stents tend to get occluded from bacterial biofilm and have the risk of falling out of the duct. Biliary SEMS offer significantly longer patency rates than 10 French plastic stents. Surgical options have shown to have greater immediate complication rates and a longer initial hospitalization than endoscopic stenting, but provide longer term palliation without the need for intervention. If ERCP is unsuccessful, surgical percutaneous transhepatic cholangiography and stent placement remains an option.[6]

References

1. Kalady MF, Peterson B, et al. Pancreatic duct strictures: identifying risk of malignancy. *Ann Surg Oncol.* 2004;11(6):581-588.
2. Inoue K, et al. Severe localized stenosis and marked dilatation of the main pancreatic duct are indicators of pancreatic cancer instead of chronic pancreatitis on endoscopic retrograde balloon pancreatography. *Gastrointest Endosc.* 2003;58(4):510-515.
3. Menges M, Lerch MM, Zeitz M. The double duct sign in patients with malignant and benign pancreatic lesions. *Gastrointest Endosc.* 2000;52:74-77.
4. Rosch T, et al. ERCP or EUS for tissue diagnosis of biliary strictures? A prospective comparative study. *Gastrointest Endosc.* 2004;60:390-396.
5. ASGE guideline: the role of ERCP in diseases of the biliary tract and the pancreas. *Gastrointest Endosc.* 2005;62: 1-8.
6. Baron TH, Mallery JS, et al. The role of endoscopy in the evaluation and treatment of patients with pancreaticobiliary malignancy. *Gastrointest Endosc.* 2003;58:643-649.

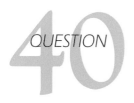
HOW SHOULD I DISCUSS THE RISKS OF POST-PROCEDURE PANCREATITIS WITH A PATIENT WHOM I AM CONSENTING FOR ENDOSCOPIC RETROGRADE CHOLANGIOPANCREATOGRAPHY? DO I REALLY HAVE TO TELL HIM HE COULD DIE?

Susan Ramdhaney, MD and Alphonso Brown, MD, MS Clin Epi

The development of pancreatitis is the most common serious iatrogenic complication following endoscopic retrograde cholangiopancreatography (ERCP). Although previously reported in the 1980s and 1990s to have an incidence of 10% to 15%, recent reports describe the risk of developing pancreatitis after an ERCP less than 3%. Accompanying this decreased incidence is a significant decrease in severity of the acute pancreatitis. The reason for this decrease is several fold—better patient selection, better technique, and improved care following the development of acute pancreatitis.

Pathogenesis of acquiring post-ERCP pancreatitis is multifactorial and includes mechanical injury from instrumentation of the pancreatic duct. Hydrostatic injury from overinjection, chemical or allergic injury from contrast medium, enzymatic injury from intestinal content, infection, and thermal injury can be graded as mild, moderate, and severe as described by Cotton et al[1] (Table 40-1).

Several factors have been identified that increase the likelihood of a patient developing pancreatitis after an ERCP. These include a history of prior post ERCP-pancreatitis, young age, female gender, sphincter of Oddi dysfunction (SOD), pancreas divisum, multiple

Table 40-1

Grading System for the Major Complications of Endoscopic Retrograde Cholangiopancreatography and Endoscopic Sphincterotomy

	Mild	*Moderate*	*Severe*
Pancreatitis	Amylase at least 3 times normal at more than 24 hours after the procedure, requiring admission or prolongation of planned admission to 2 to 3 days	Hospitalization of 4 to 10 days	Hospitalization of more than 10 days, hemorrhagic pancreatitis, phlegmon or pseudocyst, or intervention (percutaneous drainage or surgery)
Bleeding	Clinical not just endoscopic evidence of bleeding, hemoglobin drop <3 g, and no need for transfusion	Transfusion (4 units or less), no angiographic intervention or surgery	Transfusion (5 units or more) or intervention (angiographic or surgical)
Cholangitis	>38°C for 24 to 48 hours	Febrile or septic illness requiring more than 3 days of hospital treatment or endoscopic or percutaneous intervention	Septic shock or surgery
Perforation	Possible, or only very slight leak of fluid or contrast, treatable by fluids and suction for 3 days or less	Any definite perforation treated medically for 4 to 10 days	Medical treatment for more than 10 days or intervention (percutaneous or or surgical)

contrast injections into the pancreatic duct, pre-cut sphincterotomy, difficulty of cannulation, and operator dependent such as an inexperienced endoscopist. Of these risk factors, the performance of sphincter of Oddi manometry for evaluation of suspected SOD has the highest risk of inducing pancreatitis (15% to 20%). In general, the more abnormal the duct, the less likely the patient will develop post-ERCP pancreatitis.

Studies have shown that most cases of post-ERCP pancreatitis are mild or moderate with only a small number severe (0.6%). Despite the relatively common occurrence of post-ERCP pancreatitis, severe acute pancreatitis will develop in only 0.2% to 0.4% of cases and death is an extremely rare event. If death occurs, it is typically related to the co-morbid conditions of the patient, including cardiopulmonary disease.

Recently, there have been a few published studies that have shown interventions that may decrease the likelihood that an individual will develop post-ERCP pancreatitis. The most important of these are procedural, such as using wire-guided cannulation and the judicious placement of pancreatic duct stents[2] in high-risk patients such as patients with suspected SOD. The use of pure cut and then switching to blended current is currently being investigated, but initial studies are not promising. A large number of agents have also been investigated in the prophylactic use to prevent post-ERCP pancreatitis. Failed agents include antibiotics, calcitonin, glucagon, nifedipine, allopurinol,[3] secretin, intravenous glucocorticoids, gabexate mesylate, nitroglycerin,[4] and topical lidocaine with equivocal studies for agents such as ulinastatin, anticoagulation, 5-fluorouracil, somatostatin, octreotide, nonsteroidal anti-inflammatory drugs,[5,6] kinase inhibitors, and botulinum toxin which have shown to be promising in decreasing the incidence of severe acute pancreatitis following an ERCP. However, none have been consistently shown to be beneficial to routinely recommend.

Although the risk of post-ERCP pancreatitis has been significantly reduced in recent years, there is a small but real risk of death. The risk of death is more likely related to the patient's underlying medical problems, especially if cardiopulmonary disease is present, rather than the procedure itself. Careful discussion of the risks and benefits of the procedure should be carefully relayed to the patient including the risk in developing severe post-ERCP pancreatitis in comparison to the patient's underlying pancreaticobiliary disease. For example, if the patient is a young healthy woman with a normal pancreatic and biliary tree, suspected as having SOD, then the risk of developing post-ERCP pancreatitis is high, the risk of developing severe disease is high, and the risk of death may be as high as 1%, and the patient should think twice about consenting to the procedure. However, in the patient with a mass in the head of the pancreas, dilated ducts, and jaundice, the risk of post-ERCP pancreatitis, severe disease, and death from the procedure is small (<1/500 for death) compared to the patient's pancreaticobiliary disease. Our role as physicians is to adequately educate the patients and to make an educated decision if and when to perform ERCP.

References

1. Cotton PB, et al. Endoscopic sphincterotomy complications and their management: an attempt at consensus. *Gastrointest Endosc.* 1991;37:383.
2. Freeman ML. Prevention of post-ERCP pancreatitis: pharmacologic solution or patient selection and pancreatic stents? *Gastroenterology.* 2003;124(7):1977-1980.
3. Bai Y, Duowu Z, Zhaoshen L. Is indomethacin a new hope for post-ERCP pancreatitis? *Am J Gastroenterol.* 2007;102(9):2103; author reply 2103-2104.
4. Muralidharan V, Jamidar P. Pharmacologic prevention of post-ERCP pancreatitis: is nitroglycerin a sangreal? *Gastrointest Endosc.* 2006;64(3):358-360.
5. Murray B, et al. Diclofenac reduces the incidence of acute pancreatitis after endoscopic retrograde cholangiopancreatography. *Gastroenterology.* 2003;124(7):1786-1791.
6. Madanick RD, O'Loughlin CJ, Barkin JS. Diclofenac reduces the incidence of acute pancreatitis after endoscopic retrograde cholangiopancreatography. *Dig Dis Sci.* 2005;50(5):879-881.

Bibliography

Freeman ML. Understanding risk factors and avoiding complications with endoscopic retrograde cholangiopancreatography. *Curr Gastroenterol Rep.* 2003;5(2):145-153.

IN A PATIENT WITH GALLSTONE PANCREATITIS, WHEN SHOULD AN ENDOSCOPIC RETROGRADE CHOLANGIOPANCREATOGRAPHY AND/OR MAGNETIC RESONANCE CHOLANGIOPANCREATOGRAPHY BE PERFORMED PREOPERATIVELY?

Nison Badalov, MD and Robin Baradarian, MD, FACG

Gallstones are the most common cause of acute pancreatitis worldwide. The pathogenesis has not be clearly established, however, a transient obstruction of the common channel, where the pancreatic and biliary ducts merge, has stood the test of time since its first description by Opie at the turn of the century. Despite the presence of a stone transiently causing obstruction, most stones pass out of the common bile duct (CBD), out of the common channel into the duodenum, passed in the stool.

Identification of a biliary etiology of acute pancreatitis is important because recurrent episodes will occur in one-third to two-thirds of these patients in follow-up periods of as short as 3 months unless gallstones are eliminated.

Gallstones should be suspected as a cause of acute pancreatitis when there are elevations of liver chemistries (particularly alanine aminotransferase [ALT] ≥3 times the upper limit of normal). Gallstones can be documented within the CBD with accuracy similar to endoscopic retrograde cholangiopancreatography (ERCP) by endoscopic ultrasound

Figure 41-1. Endoscopic ultrasound showing stone in common bile duct.

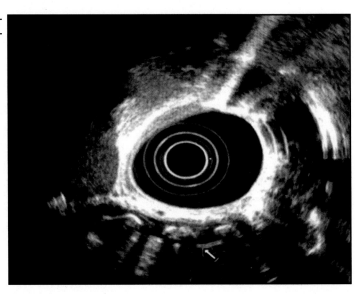

Figure 41-2. Endoscopic retrograde cholangiopancreatography showing multiple stones in common bile duct.

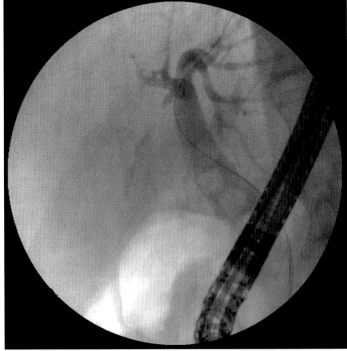

(EUS), with somewhat lower accuracy by magnetic resonance cholangiopancreatography (MRCP) (Figures 41-1 through 41-3). However, the preferred method from a cost-effective standpoint would be intraoperative cholangiography at the time of laparoscopic cholecystectomy (Table 41-1).

In general, ERCP should be performed primarily in patients with a high suspicion of bile duct stones when therapy is needed to prevent complications. Routine ERCP should be avoided in patients with low to intermediate suspicion of retained bile duct stones,

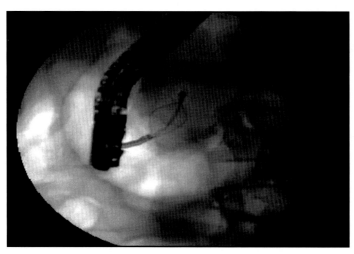

Figure 41-3. Endoscopic retrograde cholangiopancreatography showing large common bile duct stone being removed with basket lithotripsy.

Table 41-1

Indications for Endoscopic Retrograde Cholangiopancreatography, Endoscopic Ultrasound, and Magnetic Resonance Cholangiopancreatography in Patients With Acute Biliary Pancreatitis

Urgent ERCP (preferably within 24 hours of admission)
- Severe pancreatitis (organ failure)
- Suspicion of cholangitis

Elective ERCP with sphincterotomy
- Imaging study demonstrating persistent common bile duct stone
- Evolving evidence of biliary obstruction (such as rising liver chemistries)
- Poor surgical candidate for laparoscopic cholecystectomy
- Strong suspicion of bile duct stones post-cholecystectomy

EUS or MRCP to determine need for ERCP
- Clinical course not improving sufficiently to allow timely laparoscopic cholecystectomy
- and intraoperative cholangiogram
- Pregnant patient
- High-risk or difficult ERCP (eg, coagulopathy, altered surgical anatomy)
- Uncertainty regarding biliary etiology of pancreatitis

Adapted from Banks PA, Freeman ML. Practice guidelines in acute pancreatitis. *Am J Gastroenterol.* 2006;101:2379-2400.

---

who are planned to have cholecystectomy. ERCP is indicated early in the course of acute pancreatitis in patients with suspected retained bile duct stones and severe pancreatitis, complicated by cholangitis. Retained CBD stones in the setting of acute pancreatitis can lead to organ failure by causing ascending cholangitis or by causing intensification of the pancreatitis by a stone blocking the pancreatic duct.

ERCP is also indicated later, after resolution of acute pancreatitis, in patients who are poor candidates for cholecystectomy, in those who are post-cholecystectomy, and in those with strong evidence of persistent biliary obstruction. Although EUS or MRCP can be used to identify CBD stones and determine need for ERCP in clinically ambiguous situations, ERCP should not be delayed when clearly indicated due to the high probability of a CBD stone, such as a patient with severe acute pancreatitis, complicated by biliary sepsis.

The role of urgent ERCP and biliary sphincterotomy in gallstone pancreatitis has been the subject of 3 published randomized controlled studies. These studies have compared early ERCP with biliary sphincterotomy with delayed or selective ERCP. Inclusion criteria and presence of bile duct stones vary considerably among these trials. Two of the trials, but not the third, showed a significant benefit for early sphincterotomy and stone extraction, primarily in patients with severe acute pancreatitis and those with ascending cholangitis. A summary of these studies suggests that ERCP and biliary sphincterotomy is indicated (preferably within 24 hours of admission) for patients with severe biliary pancreatitis with retained CBD stones and for those with cholangitis. In addition, if during the course of biliary pancreatitis, progressive increases in serum bilirubin and other liver function tests and/or persistent dilatation of the CBD develop, suggestive of CBD obstruction by gallstones, ERCP should be performed.

In patients with mild disease, or severe disease with complete resolution of symptoms and absence of elevations of bilirubin, laparoscopic cholecystectomy with intraoperative cholangiography can be performed. Any remaining bile duct stones can be dealt with by postoperative or intraoperative ERCP, or by laparoscopic or open CBD exploration, depending on local expertise and access to referral centers in cases of unsuccessful ERCP.

The role of EUS or MRCP is not entirely clear and needs to be applied individually. These modalities can be performed to assess for the presence of bile duct stones and determine need for ERCP in patients less likely to have a CBD stone. EUS is generally considered to be the most accurate method to detect bile duct stones; sensitivity of MRCP for small bile duct stones is lower, especially for those that are impacted at the ampulla. EUS or MRCP is also useful to determine need for ERCP in patients who are pregnant or in whom ERCP would be high risk or technically difficult due to reasons such as severe coagulopathy or altered surgical anatomy. In critically ill patients, EUS can be performed at the bedside. EUS is limited by technique availability and operator dependency. MRCP is limited by variable quality, difficulty in performing this procedure in critically ill or uncooperative patients, and contraindications such as presence of pacemakers.

Bibliography

Fan ST, Lai EC, Mok FP, et al. Early treatment of acute biliary pancreatitis by endoscopic papillotomy. *N Engl J Med.* 1993;328:228-232.

Folsch UR, Nitsche R, Ludtke R, et al. Early ERCP and papillotomy compared with conservative treatment for acute biliary pancreatitis. *N Engl J Med.* 1997;336:237-242.

Makary MA, Duncan MD, Harmon JW, et al. The role of magnetic resonance cholangiography in the management of patients with gallstone pancreatitis. *Ann Surg.* 2005;241:119-124.

Mark DH, Flamm CR, Aronson N. Evidence-based assessment of diagnostic modalities for common bile duct stones. *Gastrointest Endosc.* 2002;56(Suppl 6):S190-S194.

Neoptolemos JP, London NJ, James D, Carr-Locke DL. Controlled trail of urgent endoscopic retrograde cholangio-pancreatography and endoscopic sphincterotomy versus conservative management for acute pancreatitis due to gallstones. *Lancet.* 1988;3:979-983.

Sahai AV, Mauldin PD, Marsi V, et al. Bile duct stones and laparoscopic cholecystectomy: a decision analysis to assess the roles of intraoperative cholangiography, EUS, and ERCP. *Gastrointest Endosc.* 1999;49:334-343.

Tenner S, Dubner H, Steinberg W. Predicting gallstone pancreatitis with laboratory parameters: a meta-analysis. *Am J Gastroenterol.* 1994;89:1863-1869.

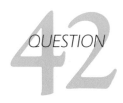

I HAVE A PATIENT WITH SUSPECTED PRIMARY SCLEROSING CHOLANGITIS. WHAT DO I NEED TO KNOW AND HOW DO I ESTABLISH THE DIAGNOSIS?

Ronald Concha-Parra, MD and Frank G. Gress, MD

Primary sclerosing cholangitis (PSC) is a chronic cholestatic liver disease characterized by inflammation, fibrosing, and destruction of the intrahepatic and/or extrahepatic biliary ducts. This disease can affect large as well as small bile ducts. Cholangiography is useful only in the detection of abnormalities of the large intrahepatic and extrahepatic bile ducts. Disease limited to the small intrahepatic ducts is diagnosed by liver biopsy.

The typical course of PSC is characterized by insidious worsening of cholestasis, advancing to portal hypertension, cirrhosis, end-stage liver disease, and death from liver failure unless transplantation is performed. PSC may have a long subclinical course and patients are frequently asymptomatic at the time of diagnosis. A median duration of 12 to 18 years from the time of diagnosis before the patient develops end-stage liver disease has been observed. Nowadays, PSC is one of the most common indications for liver transplantation with excellent post-transplant prognosis and 3-year survival rates of up to 90%.

Based on an adequate immunogenetic background, immunopathogenetic mechanisms occur, causing inflammatory changes of the bile ducts possibly triggered or intensified by infectious pathogens.[1] In PSC, perinuclear antineutrophilic autoantibody (pANCA) and antinuclear antibodies (ANA) are considered epiphenomena and are not thought to be responsible for bile duct injury.

PSC affects predominantly young and middle-aged men, with a mean age of approximately 40 years at the time of diagnosis. The majority of patients initially present with asymptomatically elevated liver enzymes. Progressive fatigue and pruritus are the most common symptoms. Jaundice, weight loss, and fever are uncommon symptoms at initial

Figure 42-1. Cholangiogram of a patient with primary sclerosing cholangitis showing widespread bile duct strictures and dilatations.

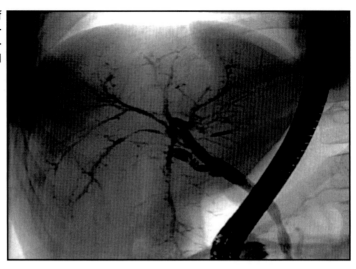

presentation. Symptoms of bacterial cholangitis (fever, abdominal pain, and jaundice) may occur in PSC patients with dominant strictures. On rare occasions, the first symptoms can reflect complications of advanced cirrhosis, such as variceal bleed and ascites. Approximately 70% to 80% of PSC patients in the United States will have or develop ulcerative colitis (UC). Furthermore, 2% to 7.5% of UC patients and 1.3% to 3.4% of Crohn's disease patients develop PSC. Inflammatory bowel disease usually precedes the development of PSC. Apart from the association with inflammatory bowel disease, more than 20% of PSC patients display at least one additional extraintestinal autoimmune feature: most frequently insulin dependent diabetes mellitus (10%), thyroid disorders (8.4%), and psoriasis (4.2%).[2]

The increase of alkaline phosphatase ranging 3 and 10 times the upper limit of normal is the hallmark of PSC. Serum alanine and aspartate aminotransferase levels are usually 2 to 3 times higher than normal levels. Serum bilirubin is elevated in 50% to 70% of PSC patients at the time of diagnosis. pANCA is present in approximately 80% of patients, but disease activity does not correlate with pANCA positivity or titer. Other auto antibodies such as ANA (20%) and antismooth muscle antibody (ASMA) (60%) may be present in 20% and 60% of patients, respectively.[3] Cholangiography is the gold standard for the diagnosis of PSC. The most frequent features include multifocal annular strictures with intervening segments of normal ducts, resulting in the typical beads-on-a-string appearance (Figure 42-1). The main pancreatic duct and the cystic duct may also be affected. Magnetic resonance cholangiopancreatography (MRCP) is a noninvasive test and avoids endoscopic retrograde cholangiopancreatography (ERCP)-related complications (eg, pancreatitis, adverse effects of contrast media associated with ERCP), but does not permit intervention such as bile duct brushing, balloon dilatation, or stent placement. MRCP is beneficial, however, in identifying patients who would require therapeutic ERCP.

The main features include concentric periductal fibrosis (onion skinning), inflammation, and bile duct proliferation alternating with ductal obliteration and ductopenia. Table 42-1 shows the Ludwig staging system for classification of PSC severity. However, liver biopsy is not necessary for diagnosis if the patient presents with typical PSC changes in cholangiography and is reserved for cases suspicious of having small duct PSC or overlap syndrome with autoimmune hepatitis.

Table 42-1

The Ludwig Staging System for Classification of Primary Sclerosing Cholangitis Severity

Stage 1—Portal stage	Portal hepatitis, bile duct abnormalities, or both; fibrosis or edema may be present; abnormalities do not exist beyond the limiting plate
Stage 2—Periportal stage	Periportal fibrosis with or without inflammation extending beyond the limiting plate; piecemeal necrosis may be present
Stage 3—Septal stage	Septal fibrosis, bridging necrosis, or both
Stage 4—Cirrhotic stage	Biliary cirrhosis

If a patient with cholestasis and UC has liver histology consistent with PSC and a normal cholangiography, small duct PSC can be assumed. An overlap syndrome of PSC and autoimmune hepatitis (AIH) is presumed in patients with PSC who also fulfill the diagnostic criteria for AIH, and this association is found in 1.4% to 8% of PSC patients.[1] Patients with immunoglobulin G4-related autoimmune pancreatitis often develop sclerosing cholangitis as an extrapancreatic manifestation. This type of sclerosing cholangitis resembles PSC in the cholangiography but unlike PSC responds well to steroid therapy.

Patients with PSC and UC who undergo proctocolectomy with a continent or conventional ileostomy may develop peristomal varices in 25% to 50% of cases.[4] Bleeding from these varices is more difficult to treat than esophageal variceal bleeding. Therapeutic approaches to this complication include liver transplantation or transjugular intrahepatic portosystemic shunt.

Pruritis is a common symptom of PSC. Osteoporosis is found in approximately 50% of PSC patients. Patients with advanced liver disease have a higher risk of developing severe osteoporosis. Early post-transplant bone loss is an additional factor predisposing to post-transplant nontraumatic fractures. Deficiencies of vitamins A, D, E, and K are frequently seen in patients with jaundice and advanced cirrhosis.

Cholangiocarcinoma is the most lethal complication of PSC. It has been reported in 4% to 20% of PSC patients. The incidence is higher in more advanced disease. A tight stricture in large caliber extrahepatic biliary ducts is a frequent finding in PSC patients and occurs in 54% to 58% of patients. It often is benign rather than malignant.

Bacteriobilia is found in the majority of PSC patients, however, bacterial cholangitis usually manifests after endoscopic intervention or biliary surgical exploration. Most infections are caused by aerobic enteric organisms. It is common in patients with a dominant stricture or bile duct stones. For PSC, the risk of post-ERCP cholangitis is significantly reduced with antibiotic prophylaxis and adequate drainage. Antibiotic prophylaxis in patients with recurrent cholangitis has not been proven to be beneficial.

Management

MEDICAL

Ursodeoxycholic acid may improve liver enzymes but does not appear to alter the course of the disease. However, it may protect against colon cancer in patients with UC. Several other drugs (corticosteroids, azathioprine, methotrexate, tacrolimus, pentoxifylline, and colchicine) have been investigated for management of PSC; however, they did not improve histology or cholangiography. Pruritus is one of the most disabling symptoms of PSC. Cholestyramine represents first-line therapy in severe cases. Other options for severe pruritus include rifampin, opioid antagonists such as oral naltrexone or intravenous naloxone. Calcium and vitamin D supplementation are recommended for osteoporosis and in selected cases biphosphonates may be indicated.

ENDOSCOPIC

Tight strictures in large caliber extrahepatic ducts may cause obstruction with an acute deterioration in liver function. These strictures may be managed endoscopically, usually by balloon dilatation followed by stent insertion to maintain patency. Dilatation appears to improve survival in patients with dominant strictures and jaundice. Short-term stenting is as effective as long-term stenting, but without the associated complication related to stent occlusion.[5] For complex strictures, particularly at the hilum, a percutaneous or combined approach may be required.

SURGICAL

Biliary resection including the hepatic duct bifurcation and postoperative transhepatic stenting or bypass remains another option for dominant strictures in noncirrhotic patients, particularly in those who fail endoscopic therapy.[6] Transplant-free survival is improved in patients treated operatively with extrahepatic duct resection. Patients with dominant strictures and equivocal cholangiocarcinoma screening results should be managed with resection if possible.

TRANSPLANTATION

Indications for liver transplantation apart from advanced cirrhosis may include intractable severe pruritus, recurrent bacterial cholangitis despite endoscopic and antibiotic therapy, extrahepatic biliary obstruction unable to be repaired surgically or endoscopically, and uncontrollable peristomal variceal bleeding. Cholangiocarcinoma has been considered a contraindication for liver transplantation because of poor outcomes related by recurrent carcinoma. Recent data, however, suggest that transplant with neoadjuvant chemoradiation used in cases of localized, node negative hilar cholangiocarcinoma may achieve better survival than conventional resection.[3] Liver transplantation in PSC patients has excellent 5-year survival rates (85% to 90%).[7] However, retransplantation rates seem to be higher than other transplant-requiring illnesses.

References

1. Weismuller TJ, Wedemeyer J, Kubicka S, Strassburg CP, Manns MP. The challenges in primary sclerosing cholangitis—aetiopathogenesis, autoimmunity, management and malignancy. *J Hepatol.* 2008;48(Suppl 1): S38-S57.
2. Saarinen S, Olerup O, Broome U. Increased frequency of autoimmune diseases in patients with primary sclerosing cholangitis. *Am J Gastroenterol.* 2000;95(11):3195-3199.
3. Silveira MG, Lindor KD. Clinical features and management of primary sclerosing cholangitis. *World J Gastroenterol.* 2008;14(21):3338-3349.
4. Gordon FD. Primary sclerosing cholangitis. *Surg Clin North Am.* 2008;88(6):1385-1407.
5. McLoughlin M, Enns R. Endoscopy in the management of primary sclerosing cholangitis. *Curr Gastroenterol Rep.* 2008;10(2):177-185.
6. Ahrendt SA. Surgical approaches to strictures in primary sclerosing cholangitis. *J Gastrointest Surg.* 2008;12(3):423-425.
7. Roberts MS, Angus DC, Bryce CL, Valenta Z, Weissfeld L. Survival after liver transplantation in the United States: a disease-specific analysis of the UNOS database. *Liver Transpl.* 2004;10(7):886-897.

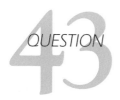

CAROLI'S DISEASE, WHAT DO I NEED TO KNOW?

Mustafa A. Tiewala, MD and Frank G. Gress, MD

Cystic lesions of the hepatobiliary system are being increasingly diagnosed. These fibropolycystic diseases involve multiple organs. They are usually inherited and occur in various combinations, consisting of polycystic liver disease, microhamartoma, congenital hepatic fibrosis, Caroli's disease, and choledochal cysts. Caroli's disease, originally described by Jacques Caroli in 1958, is a congenital disorder characterized by multiple segmental or saccular dilatations of the large intrahepatic bile ducts. Caroli's syndrome is a congenital disorder characterized by multiple segmental or saccular dilatations of the intrahepatic bile ducts associated with congenital hepatic fibrosis. The term *congenital fibrosis* refers to a unique congenital liver histology characterized by bland portal fibrosis, hyperproliferation of interlobular bile ducts within the portal areas with variable shapes and sizes of bile ducts, and preservation of the normal lobular architecture.

More than 200 cases with equal frequencies in males and females have been reported in the literature from United Kingdom, France, Japan, and the United States with Caroli's syndrome occurring more than the pure form of Caroli's disease. Symptoms appear first in adults, though childhood and neonatal cases have been reported.

The most accepted theory is related to ductal plate malformations at different levels of the intrahepatic biliary tree. The formation of the ductal plates follows the branching growth of the portal vein from the hilus to the periphery, as does the remodeling of the ductal plates which begins from the larger to smaller ducts. Thus hereditary factors influencing Caroli's syndrome influence the early embryonic development of the large intrahepatic bile duct formation as well as the development of the more proximal intralobular ducts related with congenital hepatic fibrosis.

The molecular pathogenesis is not clear. It appears to be inherited in an autosomal recessive manner, associated with autosomal recessive polycystic kidney disease

Figure 43-1. Gross pathology sections of liver show multiple saccular dilatations of intrahepatic bile ducts. Septum-like fibrovascular bundles are seen on walls of some cut sacculi (arrow) and traversing lumina of others (arrowhead). (Reprinted with permission from the *American Journal of Roentgenology.*)

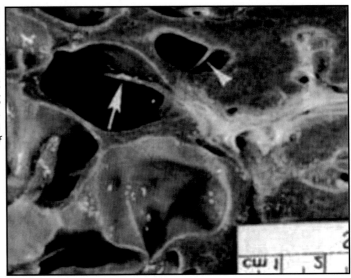

(ARPKD). The gene mapped to chromosome 6 (6p21-p12) is called the PKHD1 gene (for polycystic kidney and hepatic disease 1). It encodes for a large protein (4074 amino acids) called fibrocystin, which is involved in regulation of cell proliferation, cellular adhesions, repulsion, and ciliary function.

Mutations in two different genes, polycystic kidney disease (PKD) 1 or 2, give rise to an autosomal dominant polycystic kidney disease (ADPKD), which in rare cases is associated with Caroli's disease. Products of PKD genes (polycystin 1 and polycystin 2) are involved in cell-cell or cell-matrix interactions. Polycystin 1 is expressed in the liver including biliary system and kidney and is likely involved in embryogenesis.

As previously described, the biliary abnormality consists of segmental, saccular dilatations of the large intrahepatic bile ducts, which are in continuity with the rest of the biliary tree. The disease may be limited to 1 lobe of the liver, more commonly the left.

The dilated bile ducts are lined by biliary epithelium which may be hyperplastic and ulcerated. In Caroli's syndrome, the additional findings of congenital hepatic fibrosis characterized by bland portal fibrosis, hyperproliferation of interlobular bile ducts within the portal areas with variable shapes and sizes of bile ducts, and preservation of the normal lobular architecture are seen (Figure 43-1).

The clinical features of Caroli's syndrome are a combination of Caroli's disease (bile stasis, recurrent bouts of cholangitis, hepatolithiasis, gallbladder stones, and increased risk of cholangiocarcinoma) and those of congenital hepatic fibrosis (including portal hypertension and variceal bleeds). ARPKD frequently presents in neonates and can even be detected in utero. The symptoms may develop early or late in life. Consequences of congenital hepatic fibrosis like portal hypertension appear later in the disease process indicating that Caroli's syndrome has a progressive course. The complications of portal hypertension include ascites and esophageal varices which may present with hematemesis and malena. Patients may present with intermittent abdominal pain and pruritis associated with hyperbilirubinemia. In Caroli's disease and syndrome, the saccular dilatations predispose to bile stagnation, biliary sludge, and intraductal lithiasis, which may result in chronic abdominal pain and pancreatitis. Bacterial cholangitis occurs frequently,

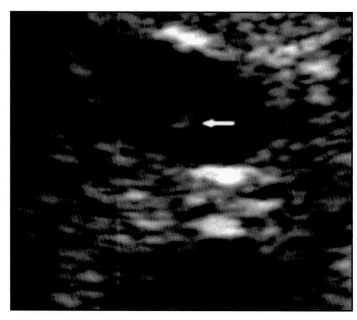

Figure 43-2. Sonogram of duct with saccular dilatation shows echogenic central dot (arrow). (Reprinted with permission from the *American Journal of Roentgenology.*)

complicated by septicemia and hepatic abscess formation. This remains the major cause of morbidity and mortality.

On examination, there may be hepatosplenomegaly from portal hypertension. Enlarged kidneys may be palpable with renal involvement. Laboratory analysis may include: alanine aminotransferase (ALT), alkaline phosphatase and bilirubin elevations, thrombocytopenia, and leukopenia if portal hypertension and hypersplenism are present. Leukocytosis may indicate cholangitis. An elevation of the blood urea nitrogen and creatinine should suggest underlying renal disease associated with this disorder. On occasion, coagulopathy may be found related to vitamin K malabsorption in cholestatic patients.

Transabdominal imaging may reveal intrahepatic cystic anechoic areas in which fibrovascular bundles, stones, and linear bridging may be seen (Figure 43-2).

Doppler sonogram may be useful by demonstrating flow within fibrovascular bundles composed of the portal vein and hepatic artery and may also be useful to follow the progression of fibrosis in patients with Caroli's syndrome.

Although there is a risk for post-endoscopic retrograde cholangiopancreatography (ERCP) pancreatitis, ERCP remains the gold standard for the evaluation of the biliary tree. The risks and benefits of this procedure need to be considered prior. In complex difficult cases of fusiform dilatation of the biliary tract, ERCP may show communication between sacculi and bile ducts and diverticulum-like sacculi of the intrahepatic biliary tree (Figure 43-3).

Computed tomography may be helpful. Although nonspecific, it may show saccular and fusiform dilatations of intrahepatic bile ducts (Figure 43-4). Fibrovascular bundles are seen as enhancing central dots (dot sign), septa, and nodules. Renal cysts may also be seen. A cirrhotic liver with signs of marked portal hypertension, which include ascites, splenomegaly, esophageal and splenic varices, and patent paraumbilical vein may be seen (Figure 43-5).

Figure 43-3. Endoscopic retrograde cholangiogram shows multiple communicating sacculi of intrahepatic biliary tree. (Reprinted with permission from the *American Journal of Roentgenology.*)

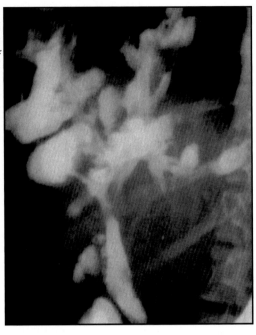

Figure 43-4. Computed tomography scan showing saccular and fusiform dilatations of intrahepatic bile ducts. Fibrovascular bundles are seen as enhancing central dots (solid arrows), septa (open arrows), and nodules (arrowheads). Renal cysts also are present. (Reprinted with permission from the *American Journal of Roentgenology.*)

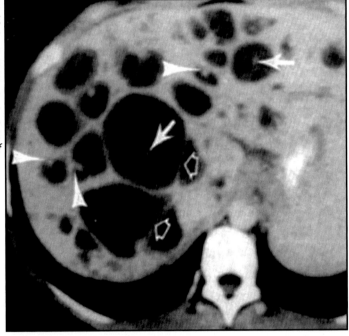

Magnetic resonance imaging is the best noninvasive imaging technique to confirm large or small cystic patterns. Combined with the use of gadolinium, it may allow visualization of the dot sign, which is very specific for malformations of the ductal plate.

A liver biopsy is not required to establish a diagnosis of Caroli's syndrome, but when obtained, it will show intrahepatic bile duct ectasia and proliferation associated with

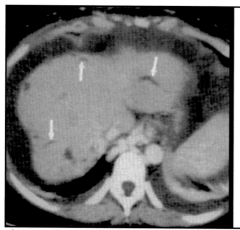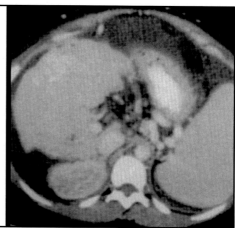

Figure 43-5. Congenital hepatic fibrosis associated with Caroli's disease. Contrast-enhanced computed tomography scans show fusiform dilatation of intrahepatic bile ducts (arrows). Liver shows cirrhotic morphology, with signs of marked portal hypertension, which include ascites, splenomegaly, esophageal and splenic varices, and patent paraumbilical vein. (Reprinted with permission from the *American Journal of Roentgenology.*)

severe periportal fibrosis, confirming the congenital hepatic fibrosis component of Caroli's syndrome. In Caroli's disease, there is only ectasia of the larger hepatic ducts. Liver biopsy may show features of cholangitis.

The differential diagnosis of cystic diseases of the liver include Caroli's syndrome, polycystic liver disease, obstructive biliary disease, primary sclerosing cholangitis, biliary papillomatosis, and choledochal cysts.

Caroli's syndrome belongs to a family of polycystic diseases, involving other organs; renal involvement is seen in 60% of cases. This manifests as dilatation of the collecting renal tubules, renal tubular ectasia, adult recessive polycystic disease, and rarely adult dominant polycystic kidney disease. Congenital heart disease, pulmonary hypertension with arteriovenous fistula, pulmonary fibrosis, and cavernomatous transformation of portal vein may be also found.

Complications of this disease include cholangitis, choledocholithiasis, hepatic abscesses, cholangiocarcinoma (seen in 7% to 14% of patients), cirrhosis, portal hypertension, and liver failure. The treatment of complications associated with Caroli's syndrome involves the use of medical, endoscopic, and surgical modalities. The medical management involves the use of antibiotics for acute cholangitis. Ursodeoxycholic acid is used in chronic cholestasis to decrease bile stasis and increase bile flow and in some cases is associated with dissolution of bile duct stones. Supportive care includes vitamin supplementation of fat-soluble vitamins in patients with chronic cholestasis. In cases of portal hypertension and varices, nonselective beta-blockers are prescribed. In the treatment of variceal hemorrhage, blood transfusions, antibiotics, somatostatin infusions, and endoscopic variceal banding are required. Transjugular intrahepatic porto-systemic shunts, surgical port-caval shunts are considered in patients not responsive to band ligation or sclerotherapy.

Endoscopic management for drainage of bile involves the use of ERCP with possible sphincterotomy and stone removal. Drainage during percutaneous transhepatic cholangiography is another option. Imaging modalities are used to plan surgical treatment. If one lobe of the liver is involved, then hepatic resection is curative. Internal bypass procedures like choledochojejunostomy and Roux-en-Y hepaticojejunostomy are used for diffuse disease. Liver or dual liver-kidney transplantation is curative in both Caroli's disease and Caroli's syndrome with kidney involvement. Since the disease has an autosomal recessive transmission, family genetic counseling is important.

The prognosis is variable depending upon the severity of symptoms and other organs involved. Increased morbidity is associated with recurrent cholangitis. There is an increased risk of 7% to 14% of developing cholangiocarcinoma. Amyloidosis has been seen in chronic or recurrent cholangitis. Liver transplantation offers a curative option in refractory disease.

Bibliography

Mesleh M, Deziel DJ. Bile duct cysts. *Surg Clin North Am.* 2008;88:1369-1384.

Miller WJ, Sechtin AG, Campbell WL, Pieters PC. Imaging findings in Caroli's disease. *American Journal of Roentgenology.* 1995;165:333-337.

Summerfield JA, Nagafuchi Y, Sherlock S, Cadafalch J, Scheuer PJ. Hepatobiliary fibroploycystic diseases. A clinical and histological review of 51 patients. *J Hepatol.* 1986;2(2):141-156.

Waechter FL, Sampaio JA, Pinto RD, et al. The role of liver transplantation in patient's with Caroli's disease. *Hepatogastroenterology.* 2001;48(39):672-674.

Yonem O, Bayraktar Y. Clinical characteristics of Caroli's syndrome. *World J Gastroenterol.* 2007;13(13):1934-1937.

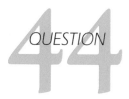
CHOLEDOCHAL CYST, WHAT TO DO? WATCH, IGNORE, OR OPERATE?

Yuriy Tsirlin, MD and Frank G. Gress, MD

Choledochal cysts are fairly rare findings of dilated extra- and/or intrahepatic sites. They are considered to be a disease of childhood and about 60% to 80% are diagnosed before the age of 10. However, at least 20% will go undiagnosed all the way into adulthood. The incidence of cystic dilatation of biliary ducts varies greatly among reports, anywhere from 1:100,000 to 150,000 to 1:2,000,000 with a female to male predominance of 3 to 4:1. The prevalence of this entity is higher in Eastern Asian countries, especially Japan; the reason for this discrepancy is unclear.

No clear etiology for bile duct cysts have been agreed on by the scientific community. It is believed to be of both congenital and acquired types. Multiple theories, however, have been proposed to explain this entity. The most favored hypothesis has been dubbed as anomalous pancreaticobiliary junction (APBJ), also called pancreaticobiliary maljunction, which is a rare congenital condition where the junction between pancreatic and common bile duct (CBD) lies outside of the duodenal wall with a long common channel, often over 1 to 2 cm (Figure 44-1). APBJ can further be classified as having acute or right angle of junction. It is theorized that this kind of anatomical connection allows free backflow of pancreatic juice into the biliary system, where activation of pancreatic proteolytic enzymes results in damage of biliary epithelium, inflammation, ductal distention, and cyst formation. This theory has been partially supported by some animal studies and by the fact that APBJ has been reported in 60% to 96% of patients with biliary cysts. This, however, does not explain the rest of the patients with bile duct cysts. Other ideas include unequal proliferation of embryologic biliary epithelial cells during development before cannulation is complete resulting in cyst formation. It has also been speculated that distal obstruction of the CBD may play a role in pathogenesis, which has been supported by some animal studies where ligation of distal duct causes formation of cysts, though this is more likely in prenatal or neonatal period as similar obstruction in adults causes dilatation of the whole biliary tree. Similar to distal obstruction, such factors as sphincter of Oddi dysmotility or oligoganglionosis of the distal CBD producing "functional" obstruction have been proposed as pathogenic factors. Infectious (ie, viral) etiology has also been proposed to play a role, especially in view of the fact that RNA of the reovirus has been isolated from biliary tissues of infants with biliary obstruction and choledochal cysts. Though no definitive hereditary pattern has been established, some familial occurrence of cysts has been described; considering increased incidence of these anomalies in Asian countries, a genetic or environmental predisposition has been contemplated to exist.

In 1959, Alonso-Lej[1] analyzed 96 cases of choledochal cysts and came up with a classification system with 3 categories. In 1977, the system was refined by Todani[2] to include 5 major classes; this was further enhanced by the same group[3] in 2003 to include presence of APBJ.

Type I is most commonly reported, comprises 50% to 85%, and is described as dilatation of the CBD, which may be cystic, focal, or fusiform. The second most common type is IVA, which is defined as both intra- and extrahepatic dilatation of the biliary tree. The remaining types are much rarer with only occasional reports being published; type II is the rarest (Table 44-1).

The classical presentation of choledochal cysts, usually described as a triad of jaundice, pain, and an abdominal mass, is found in only 11% to 63% and is much more common in children than adults. In older patients, children over age of 2 and especially so in adults, symptoms are vaguer, usually nothing more than some abdominal discomfort or pain in the right upper quadrant. Abdominal pain, whether or not accompanied by jaundice, will usually prompt some type of abdominal imaging, which will result in suspected diagnosis. In adults, however, timing of diagnosis from onset of symptoms may be prolonged, with average duration quoted as 6 years; many of these patients are thought to have gallstones or cholecystitis, and anywhere from 10% to 50% will undergo some surgical procedure (ie, cholecystectomy) prior to correct diagnosis. There are no specific laboratory tests to diagnose bile duct cysts and if abnormalities are present, they are more likely to signify complications of the anomaly such as pancreatitis, cholecystitis, and in chronic cases even advanced liver disease, such as biliary cirrhosis. It is important to note that lithiasis is fairly common in patients with choledochal cysts; stones can occur in the gallbladder, in the cysts themselves, and in the hepatic ducts proximal to stenotic areas. Cystic rupture presenting with resulting biliary peritonitis has been rarely reported.

Cross-sectional imaging such as ultrasound or computed tomography (CT) scan can often suggest presence of choledochal cyst. Cholangiography has long been considered to be the best test to evaluate biliary anatomy and can be done intraoperatively, percuteniously, or endoscopically, each having its own pros and cons. With recent advances in technology, magnetic resonance cholangiopancreatography (MRCP) has mostly replaced other more invasive tests for diagnostic purposes since its accuracy closely approaches the direct ductal imaging of endoscopic retrograde cholangiopancreatography (ERCP). The newer models of multidetector CT scanners have also proven to be useful and fairly accurate diagnostic modalities.

It has been well described that choledochal cysts carry an increased incidence of malignancy, usually of adenocarcinoma type, although occasional squamous cell and anaplastic cell carcinomas have been discovered. Generally, cancer originates in the pos-

Table 44-1
Classification of Choledochal Cysts*

Type IA	Cystic dilatation of CBD associated with APBJ	
Type IB	Segmental dilatation of CBD without APBJ	
Type IC	Associated with APBJ and has fusiform, diffuse dilatation of the CBD often continuous into intrahepatic ducts	
Type II	True diverticulum of the extrahepatic bile duct, located proximal to the duodenum	
Type III	Cystic dilatation limited to the intraduodenal portion of the distal CBD, also known as choledochocele	
Type IIIA	Bile duct and pancreatic duct enter the choledochocele, which then drains into the duodenum at a separate orifice	
Type IIIB	Diverticulum of the intraduodenal bile duct or common channel	
Type IVA	Multiple intrahepatic and extrahepatic cystic dilatations	
Type IVB	Multiple extrahepatic dilatations without intrahepatic involvement	
Type V	Isolated or multiple intrahepatic dilatations without extrahepatic involvement—Caroli's disease	

*Based on Todani.
APBJ=anomalous pancreaticobiliary junction, CBD=common bile duct.
Illustrations by Shana Hyvat.

terior wall of the cyst, though areas outside of the cyst can also be involved. The incidence of carcinoma has been reported anywhere from 2.5% to 26% and though some believe that this is highly overestimated, it is obvious that rates of malignancy in patients with choledochal cysts are at least 20 to 30 times more than that in the general population. Cancers are more likely to occur in adults but reports of carcinoma findings in children 10 and under have been published. The risk of developing cancer in children under 10 is about 0.7%; it increases to 6.8% in the second decade of life and to 14.3% in those over age 20. Types I and IV cysts are the best studied in terms of cancer risk and in fact have the most

Figure 44-1. Adenocarcinoma in bile duct cyst. Endoscopic retrograde cholangiopancreatography demonstrates type I cyst with large irregular filling defect. (Reprinted with permission from Mesleh M, Deziel DJ. Bile duct cysts. *Surg Clin North Am.* 2008;88:1369-1384.)

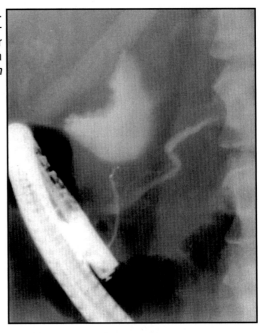

Figure 44-2. Type III bile duct cyst (choledochocele). (Reprinted with permission from Mesleh M, Deziel DJ. Bile duct cysts. *Surg Clin North Am.* 2008;88:1369-1384.)

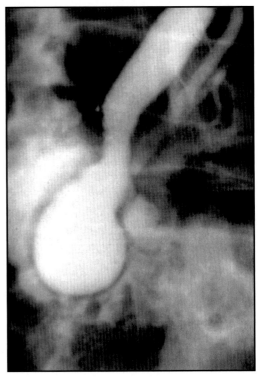

preponderance for such (in that particular order) (Figure 44-1). Type III is considered to be least common in terms of developing malignancy (Figure 44-2).

A significant association of APBJ with malignancy has been noted; it even appears that presence of pancreatobiliary maljunction is more important than choledochal cyst itself. In fact, in patients with choledochal cysts, presence of APBJ appears to increase risk of malignancy 10-fold. It is important to note that presence of APBJ carries risk of malignancy even without presence of choledochal cyst, but the location of neoplasm seems to differ. In patients without bile duct cyst but with finding of APBJ, neoplasm occurs exclusively in the gallbladder, while in those with cystic malformation, malignancy is usually inside the cyst, though gallbladder cancer can still occur. The resulting theory based on these findings rests on the idea that carcinogenic effect may be caused by the reflux of pancreatic juices that biliary mucosa is exposed to. It has been shown that histological changes inside the biliary cyst progress with age from epithelial denudement, to inflammatory infiltrates, glandular metaplasia, and, ultimately, malignancy. It is theorized that exposure of the bile duct cells to pancreatic enzymes promotes or accelerates this carcinogenic progression; given this knowledge, it stands to presume that malignancy is likely to originate in areas of low bile flow, which allows greater exposure to pancreatic enzymes. In patients with choledochal cysts, this area is inside the cyst, since it is closer to the pancreatic duct. In the absence of the cyst, this area is inside gallbladder, which explains predisposition for such cancer in these patients.

In the not-so-distant past (1970s), a cholecystenterostomy was considered a procedure of choice for management of choledochal cysts. Over time, however, due to high risk of long-term complications after this procedure and especially due to the risk of malignant transformation, cyst excision with hepaticoenterostomy has become the norm. This comes from the fact that among those patients treated with cystenterostomy internal drainage procedure, 70% needed to be reoperated because of complications such as cholangitis and hepatolithiasis; risk of malignancy in the cystic remnant by itself warrants reoperation.

Therefore, resection of the cyst and gallbladder with Roux-en-Y choledocho- or hepaticojejunostomy is the current surgical approach, with the latter reported to have less long-term stricturing complications. In type I cysts, resection of the intrapancreatic portion of the distal bile duct is required as well, and excision sample should be all the way to just below hepatic bifurcation. Careful examination is taken to exclude any further involvement. Sample is examined histologically for presence of malignancy.

Type II cysts can be managed by simple excision of the cyst and closure of the CBD defect. Cholecystectomy is recommended at the same time.

Type III cysts are the most controversial in regards to management as some would recommend a minimally invasive approach of simple sphincterotomy and drainage, which is an attractive recommendation since it can be done endoscopically. However, though risk of malignant transformation is lowest in this class, periampulary cancers have been reported inside the choledochocele, and in one study was in 3 out of 11 patients. Therefore, in a good surgical candidate, a complete resection of type III cyst is still advised and can be done by using a less invasive transduodenal surgical approach.

Type IV, both A and B, cysts warrant resection of the extrahepatic biliary tree; resection of intrahepatics are obviously not as simple and decision must be made based on disease state, such as bilobar involvement, presence of stones, strictures, and/or cirrhosis. Some also recommend partial hepatectomy in type IVA cysts if they are localized to the left lobe, since intrahepatics are often involved in malignant transformation in this type of disease.

Type V cysts (Caroli's disease), similar to type IVA, present a challenge, in that excision of all intrahepatic dilatations is not feasible and in diffuse disease treatment consists of surveillance and supportive measures in cases of biliary cirrhosis or portal hypertension. Once these or other signs of liver failure develop, liver transplantation may be an option. Also, similar to type IVA, in cases where disease is localized to a single lobe, resection of such may be undertaken.

In summary, choledochal cysts are rare and may be congenital or acquired. Most cases are diagnosed in young children, though at least 20% go undiagnosed into adulthood and this number is increasing as more incidental findings are noted on imaging done for other reasons. Clinical presentation is usually vague and nonspecific and good imaging is imperative to outline anatomy; MRCP is currently the study of choice for a suspected bile duct cyst. Long-term effects of choledochal cysts include lithiasis, cholangitis, pancreatitis, and biliary cirrhosis as well increased risk of malignancy with types I and IVA having the most risk. Treatment generally involves surgical excision of the duct and hepaticoenterostomy to regain biliary continuity; this should be done as soon as diagnosis is made to try to prevent long-term effects of the disease. It is important to note that surgery reduces but does not eliminate the risk of malignancy. In patients where surgery is not feasible, supportive measures and lifelong surveillance for malignancy should be undertaken. In those with signs and symptoms of liver failure, urgent transplant evaluation is needed.

References

1. Alonso-Lej F, Rever WB Jr, Pessagno DJ. Congenital choledochal cyst, with a report of 2, and an analysis of 94, cases. *Int Abstr Surg.* 1959;108(1):1-30.
2. Todani T, et al. Congenital bile duct cysts: classification, operative procedures, and review of thirty-seven casess including cancer arising from choledochal cyst. *Am J Surg.* 1977;134:263-269.
3. Todani T, et al. Classification of congenital biliary cystic disease: special reference to typ Ic and IVA cysts with primary ductal stricture. *J Hepatobiliary Pancreat Surg.* 2003;10:340-344.

Bibliography

Chatila R, Andersen DK, Topazian M. Endoscopic resection of a choledochocele. *Gastrointest Endosc.* 1999;50(4):578-580.

Komi N, Takehara H, Kunitomo K, et al. Does the type of anomalous arrangement of pancreaticobiliary ducts influence the surgery and prognosis of choledochal cysts? *J Pediatr Surg.* 1992;27(6):728-731.

Mesleh M, Deziel DJ. Bile duct cysts. *Surg Clin North Am.* 2008;88:1369-1384.

Metcalfe MS, Wemyss-Holden SA, Maddern GJ. Management dilemmas with choledochal cysts. *Arch Surg.* 2003;138:333-339.

Savader SJ, Benenati JF, et al. Choledochal cyts: classification and cholangeographic appearance. *American Journal of Roentgenology.* 1991;156:327-331.

Soreide K, Korner H, Havnen J, Soreide JA. Bile duct cysts in adults. *Br J Surg.* 2004;91:1538-1548.

Soreide K, Soreide JA. Bile duct cysts as precursors to biliary tract cancer. *Ann Surg Oncol.* 2007;14:1200-1211.

Stain SC, Guthrie CR, Yellin AE, Donovan AJ. Choledochal cyst in the adult. *Ann Surg.* 1995;222(2):128-133.

Visser BC, et al. Congenital choledochal cysts in adults. *Arch Surg.* 2004;139:855-862.

Weyant MJ, Maluccio MA, Choledochal cysts in adults: a report of two cases and review of literature. *Am J Gastroenterol.* 1998;93:2580-2583.

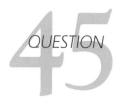

WHAT TO DO IN A PATIENT SUSPECTED OF HAVING CHOLANGIOCARCINOMA?

Hui Hing (Jack) Tin, MD and Robin Baradarian, MD, FACG

Cholangiocarcinoma is a rare malignant tumor arising from the biliary epithelium. Despite advances in diagnostic techniques during the past decade, cholangiocarcinoma is usually encountered at an advanced stage due to the late presentation of symptoms. Clinical presentation of cholangiocarcinoma depends in part on the location of the tumor within the biliary system. Intrahepatic cholangiocarcinoma presents with nonspecific symptoms including malaise, weight lost, abdominal pain, and diminished appetite and rarely as an incidental abdominal mass. Patients with extrahepatic cholangiocarcinoma present with painless jaundice, pruritis, dark urine, pale stools, and occasionally cholangitis.[1]

Early diagnosis with tissue confirmation and staging of the disease is important as only surgical resection is curative. Classification of cholangiocarcinoma is based on intrahepatic, extrahepatic, and hilar location. The Bismuth-Corlette classification is used for staging (Figure 45-1). Liver biochemical tests reflective of obstruction of the bile duct but are of limited use in differentiating among conditions. Although one large series suggests a serum carcinoembryonic antigen (CEA) level of greater than 5 ng/mL had a sensitivity and specificity of 68% and 82%, respectively, in general a serum CEA level is neither sensitive nor specific to diagnose cholangiocarcinoma. However, in the setting of a bile duct obstruction, a bile CEA level of greater than 5-fold is suggestive of cholangiocarcinoma compared to benign strictures.

Serum CA 19-9 may be more useful. CA 19-9 is widely used particularly for detecting cholangiocarcinoma in patients with primary sclerosing cholangitis (PSC). The optimal cut-off valve that best discriminates between benign or malignant biliary tract disease is influenced by the presence of cholangitis and cholestasis. In patients without either, a level of 129 U/mL has a 79% sensitivity and 99% specificity. While in patients with either

Figure 45-1. Bismuth-Corlette classification of hilar cholangiocarcinoma. Type I hilar cholangiocarcinoma involves only the common hepatic duct, distal to the confluence of the left and right hepatic ducts (biliary confluence). Type II involves the biliary confluence. Type IIIA affects the right hepatic duct in addition to the biliary confluence, and Type IIIB involves the left hepatic duct in addition to the biliary confluence. Type IV tumors either involve both the right and left hepatic ducts in addition to the biliary confluence or are multifocal.

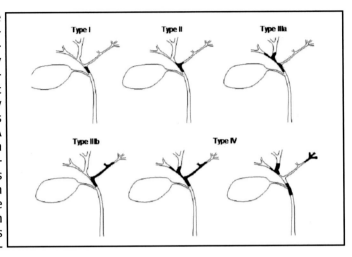

condition, a cut-off of greater than 300 U/mL was optimal for increased specificity of 87% but sensitivity of 41%. Optimal cut-off for cholangiocarcinoma in patients with PSC is greater than 400 U/mL.

Radiologic and imaging studies are essential in establishing the cause of jaundice, whether bile duct strictures are benign or malignant, and planning management in patients with suspected cholangiocarcinoma. Imaging modalities include ultrasound (US), computed tomography (CT), magnetic resonance imaging (MRI), magnetic resonance cholangiopancreatography (MRCP), angiography, scintigraphy, and positron emission tomography (PET). Endoscopic modalities for diagnosis include endoscopic retrograde cholangiopancreatography (ERCP) with or without choledochoscopy and biopsy or brushing and endoscopic ultrasound (EUS) with fine needle aspiration.

US is the image of choice for diagnosis of obstructive jaundice and demonstrates ductal obstruction in 89%, and its sensitivity for localizing the site of obstruction was 94%. Ductal dilatation appears proximal to the level of the obstruction. The exact location of the tumor can be suggested if there is an abrupt change in ductal diameter and there is an absence of stones. Another important feature of diagnostic US is the ability to evaluate vascular involvement. In one report, preoperative US detected 13 of 16 cases involving the hepatic vein (81% sensitivity, 97% specificity, and 87% positive predictive value), and in another case series, 38 of 41 patients were found to have vascular involvement giving a sensitivity of 93%, specificity 99%, positive and negative predictive value of 98%.

CT permits the identification of bile duct dilatation and assessment for metastases in the the hepatic parenchyma, lymph nodes, and distant tissues.[2] However, its ability to establish the extent of intraductal tumor spread and resectability is limited even with multiphasic CT. In one study, a report of 29 patients with histological-proven hilar cholangiocarcinoma, resectability was correctly predicted in only 60% and N2 nodal disease for CT is only 50%. With multidetector CT, the accuracy in predicting resectability has improved to 74.5% to 91.7%.

MRCP is an excellent noninvasive technique for evaluating the intrahepatic and extrahepatic bile ducts and the pancreatic ducts. It allows 3-dimensional imaging of the biliary tree and vascular structures. Cholangiocarcinoma appear as hypointense lesions

Table 45-1
Tissue or Cytologic Diagnosis of Cholangiocarcinoma

	Sensitivity	*Specificity*	*PPV*	*NPV*	*Accuracy*
ERCP/cholangiogram with brushings	35%–75%	97%–100%	96%–100%	12.5%–44%	56%–75.9%
ERCP with transpapillary biopsy	43%–81%	97%–100%	97%–100%	41%–67%	58%–86%
EUS with fine needle biopsy	86%	100%	100%	57%	88%

ERCP=endoscopic retrograde cholangiopancreatography, EUS=endoscopic ultrasound, NPV=negative predictive value, PPV=positive predictive value.

Table 45-2
Comparison of Imaging Methods for the Detection of Cholangiocarcinoma

Size of Cholangiocarcinoma	*Endoscopic Ultrasound*	*Ultrasound*	*Computed Tomography*
<2.0 cm	90%	60%	70%
>2.0 cm	100%	89%	89%
All tumors	95%	74%	79%

on T1-weighted images that are hyperintense on T2-weighted images. MRCP provides information about disease extent and potential resectability that is at least comparable to that obtained using CT, cholangiography, and angiography.

PET scan permits visualization of the cholangiocarcinomas because of high glucose uptake of the bile duct epithelium. Its more important role is the identification of occult metastases. In one series, PET led to a change in surgical management in 11 of 36 patients because of suspected metastasis.

Cholangiography performed either by percutaneous transhepatic cholangiography (PTC) or ERCP were previously done before the development of MRCP although distant or local spread cannot be visualized. Brushings or biopsies can be obtained in ERCP or PTC. The brushings can be analyzed cytologically but has low negative predictive value. Biopsy of stricture or lesions with cholangioscope increases the sensitivity only 35% to 75% to 43% to 81%.

Endoscopic ultrasound (EUS) can visualize the local extent of the primary tumor and status of regional lymph nodes. EUS-guided fine needle biopsy of tumors and enlarged nodes can also be performed, which has better sensitivity than ERCP with brushings (Table 45-1). In one study of detection of pancreatobiliary cancer, EUS was found to be superior to transabdominal ultrasound, CT, and angiography (Table 45-2).[3]

Figure 45-2. Cholangiocarcinoma identified at endoscopic retrograde cholangiopancreatography in a patient with obstructive jaundice. CA 19-9 was 1100. Diagnosis confirmed by cytology. Access for placement of silicone-coated stent.

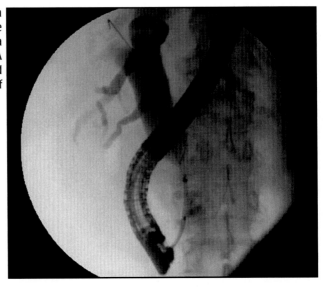

Figure 45-3. Example of a silicone-coated stent used for decompression of the bile duct for palliative care.

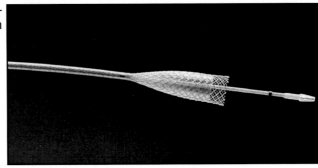

When a diagnosis of cholangiocarcinoma is confirmed at biopsy or highly likely due to a patient's overall clinical, laboratory, and radiologic findings, attention has to be paid to potential resectability of the lesion since surgery therapy offers the best potential curative for both intrahepatic and extrahepatic cholangiocarcinomas. Early stage intrahepatic cholangiocarcinoma is generally treated with resection alone. With early stage extrahepatic cholangiocarcinoma, pancreatoduodenectomy is the treatment of choice. Surgical treatment of perihilar cholangiocarcinoma depends on the Bismuth-Corlette classification (see Figure 45-1). Types I and II tumors are recommended for en bloc resection of the extrahepatic bile ducts and gallbladder, regional lymphadenectomy, and Roux-en-Y hepaticojejunostomy. Types II and III tumors may need caudate lobectomy as well. Type IV is generally unresectable.[4]

Therapy for unresectable disease may include biliary drainage or stenting, biliary ablation or intraluminal brachytherapy, and photodynamic therapy (Figures 45-2 and 45-3). Chemotherapy and radiation therapy have limited benefit. If considered, patients should be referred to tertiary centers. In advanced disease, due to the progressive nature of the disease, palliative therapy, comfort care, and hospice should be considered.

References

1. De Groen PC, Gores GJ, LaRusso NF, et al. Biliary tract cancers. *N Engl J Med.* 1999;341:1368.
2. Tajiri T, Yoshida H, Mamada Y, et al. Diagnosis and initial management of cholangiocarcinoma with obstructive jaundice. *World J Gastroenterol.* 2008;14(19):3000-3005.
3. Sugiyama M, Atomi Y, Wada N, et al. A prospective comparison with bile and brush cytology. *Am J Gastroenterol.* 1996;91:465.
4. Malhi H. Cholangiocarcinoma: modern advances in understanding a deadly old disease. *J Hepatol.* 2006; 45(6):856-867.

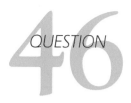

HOW OFTEN SHOULD I PERFORM ENDOSCOPIC RETROGRADE CHOLANGIOPANCREATOGRAPHY IN ORDER TO RETAIN AN ADEQUATE LEVEL OF SKILL?

Susan Ramdhaney, MD and Alphonso Brown, MD, MS Clin Epi

The use of endoscopic retrograde cholangiopancreatography (ERCP) today has moved from diagnostic and therapeutic to predominantly therapeutic with the advent of magnetic resonance cholangiopancreatography (MRCP). To perform basic therapeutic ERCP expertly, one must possess proficiency in performing sphincterotomy and stent placement of the common bile duct and pancreatic duct, stone removal using a variety of balloons and baskets, balloon dilatation of strictures, and tissue sampling using brushes and biopsy forceps. Advanced endoscopists also command knowledge of complicated bile duct stone management such as mechanical, electrohydraulic, laser, extracorporeal, and shock wave lithotripsy; pancreatic duct stone and stricture management; pseudocyst drainage; ampullectomy; and other miscellaneous procedures such as photodynamic therapy, brachytherapy, minor papillary therapy, needle-knife sphincterotomy, and rendezvous techniques. These endoscopists must be able to recognize and deal with the potential complications of such procedures: pancreatitis, bleeding, cholangitis, and perforation and should be familiar with and able to perform diagnostic techniques such as sphincter of Oddi manometry, cholangioscopy, pancreatoscopy, and interductal ultrasound.

To date, there is no definitive evidence-based criteria for ascertaining when clinical competence is achieved for ERCP. Although there are guidelines for determining the number of procedures required for credentialing, this does not necessarily indicate competency, especially since this may vary depending on the technicality of the procedure and the experience of the endoscopist.

Guidelines from Gastroenterology Core Curriculum 1996 indicate that a minimum number of procedures to be completed for competency include 100 ERCPs including 25 therapeutic cases (20 sphincterotomies and 5 stent placements), along with other earlier studies proposing the same number of procedures needed.[1] As the techniques advance, some published studies have suggested that increased numbers are required. Jowell et al[2] assessed procedural competence by evaluating the number of supervised ERCPs that physicians need to perform to achieve competence (0.8 probability of successfully completing specific technical components of ERCP). By grading 17 gastroenterology fellows performing consecutive 1796 ERCPs, they determined that at least 180 ERCPs were required to be considered competent that would enable them to practice in an unsupervised setting and that they needed to perform 50 or more per year in order to maintain technical expertise and competence. Since then other studies suggest a minimum of 200 procedures is sufficient to achieve competency[3] and now, American Society for Gastrointestinal Endoscopy (ASGE) guidelines for *ERCP Core Curriculum* mentions that seldom can trainees achieve adequate selection cannulation rates even after 200 procedures have been performed and proposes that a grading system be applied according to the degree of difficulty to gauge competency (Table 46-1). Verma et al[4] uses deep cannulation of the common bile duct as a measure of competence. They showed that successful cannulation rate increased from 43% in the beginning of training to 80% or greater after 350 to 400 supervised procedures. The success rate continued to improve post-training with an aggregated success rate of greater than 96% for the next 300 procedures performed as an independent operator.

ASGE guidelines for methods of granting hospital privileges to perform gastrointestinal endoscopy indicates that the published numbers are not adequate to achieve competency and emphasizes the need to use objective criteria of skill, rather than an arbitrary number or procedures performed when granting privileges for endoscopic procedures. Subsequent studies have shown that maintenance of ERCP competence and technical expertise is directly related to volume of patients seen.[5,6]

Regardless of the number of procedures needed, ASGE clearly outlines in its guidelines for renewal of endoscopic privileges that maintaining competence is important since procedural dexterity optimizes patient safety and comfort and that performing a procedure infrequently may lead to missed or inappropriate diagnosis. In addition, they propose that changes in equipment through upgrade necessitate familiarity, the endoscopic recognition of lesions may improve over time, and endoscopic therapy continues to undergo evaluation and evolution, and these should be re-evaluated and monitored on a constant basis.

The bottom line is that although performing a minimum number of 180 to 200 ERCPs appears reasonable to learn the technique, the art of the skill can only be developed as per the endoscopist's discretion who should be the ultimate judge in determining if he or she can expertly diagnose and treat biliary disease via ERCP with minimal complications and to the patient's overall benefit.

Table 46-1
Endoscopic Retrograde Cholangiopancreatography Degree of Difficulty Grades*

	Biliary Procedures	*Pancreatic Procedures*
Grade 1	Diagnostic cholangiogram Biliary brush cytology Standard sphincterotomy ± Removal stones <10 mm Stricture dilatation/stent/ NBD for extrahepatic stricture of bile leak	Diagnostic pancreatogram Pancreatic cytology
Grade 2	Diagnostic cholangiogram with BII anatomy Removal of CBD stones >10 mm Stricture dilatation/stent/NBD for hilar tumors or benign intrahepatic strictures	Diagnostic pancreatogram with BII anatomy Minor papilla cannulation
Grade 3	Sphincter of Oddi manometry Cholangioscopy Any therapy with BII anatomy Removal of intrahepatic stones or any stones with lithotripsy	Sphincter of Oddi manometry Pancreatoscopy All pancreatic therapy, including pseudocyst drainage

BII=Bilroth II, CBD=common bile duct, NBD=nasobiliary drain.
*Johanson JF, Cooper G, Eisen GM, et al. Quality assessment of ERCP. Endoscopic retrograde cholangiopacreatography. *Gastrointest Endosc*. 2002;56:165-169.
This table is modified from the grading system proposed by Schutz SM, Abbott RM. Grading ERCPs by degree of difficulty: a new concept to produce more meaningful outcome data. *Gastrointest Endosc*. 2000;51:535-539.

References

1. Garciá Lizcano J, González Martın JA. Training in cannulation of bile duct using endoscopic retrograde cholangiopancreatography. *Gastrointest Endosc*. 2000;58:345-349.
2. Jowell PS, Baillie J, Branch MS, et al. Quantitative assessment of procedural competence: a prospective study of training in endoscopic retrograde cholangiopancreatography. *Ann Intern Med*. 1996;983-989.
3. Garcia-Cano J. 200 supervised procedures: the minimum threshold number for competency in performing endoscopic retrograde cholangiopancreatography. *Surg Endosc*. 2007;21(7):1254-1255.
4. Verma D, Gostot CT, Petersen B, Levy M, Baron T, Adler D. Establishing a true assessment of endoscopic competence in ERCP during training and beyond: a single-operator learning curve for deep biliary cannulation in patients with native papillary anatomy. *Gastrointest Endosc*. 2007;65(3):394-400.
5. Kowalski T, Kanchana T, Pungpapong S. Perceptions of gastroenterology fellows regarding ERCP competency and training. *Gastrointest Endosc*. 2003;58(3):345-349.
6. Sedlack R, Petersen B, Binmoeller K, et al. A direct comparison of ERCP teaching models. *Gastrointest Endosc*. 2003;57(7):886-890.

SECTION VII

MISCELLANEOUS

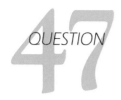

WHAT IS THE BEST APPROACH TO THE PATIENT WITH SUSPECTED SPHINCTER OF ODDI DYSFUNCTION?

Nison Badalov, MD and Scott Tenner, MD, MPH

The single most important aspect of treating a patient suspected of having sphincter of Oddi dysfunction (SOD) is to be certain of the diagnosis. There are 3 types of SOD (Table 47-1). Although the sphincter may be found to be hypertensive in these patients on manometry, differences in the clinical presentation exist and correlate with the likelihood of the diagnosis. While a patient with recurrent attacks of pancreatitis or biliary-like pain who also presents with a dilated common bile duct (CBD) and abnormal liver function tests, in the absence of obvious tumor, cholelithiasis, and choledocholithiasis, has the most evidence as having the disease (type I SOD), the patient with pain in the absence of objective findings may have irritable bowel syndrome and a conservative approach would be recommended (type III).

The use of manometry alone to establish the diagnosis has the least evidence to support any intervention. Due to the high rate of complications, including pancreatitis, bleeding, and perforation, the commonly accepted intervention for SOD, sphincterotomy, should only be used if the diagnosis is with a high degree of certainty (in patients with type I or II SOD).

At times referred to as hypertensive or fibrotic SOD, SOD causes diminished transsphincteric flow of bile and/or pancreatic juice due to either organic obstruction (stenosis) or functional obstruction (dysmotility). SOD often causes recurrent pain with or without abnormalities of either hepatic/pancreatic profiles as well as duct dilatation. It is thought that SOD causes pancreatitis as a result of bile reflux into the pancreatic duct or from pancreatic duct outflow obstruction. SOD is considered to cause up to one-third of all cases of idiopathic pancreatitis. In order to diagnose SOD, one often needs to perform sphincter of Oddi manometry (SOM). The diagnostic gold standard is a water-perfused catheter system that can be inserted into the CBD or pancreatic duct with the positive finding

---

Table 47-1

Accuracy of Sphincter of Oddi Dysfunction as a Cause of Acute Recurrent Pancreatitis

Type I

    1. Elevation of pancreatic enzymes (>1.5 times normal) amylase and/or lipase

    2. Dilated pancreatic duct (>6 mm head, >5 mm body)

    3. Delayed drainage of contrast (>9 minutes)

Type II

    One or two of the above

Type III

    None of the above

Accuracy: Type I: 92%, Type II: 58%, Type III: 35%.

---

being a hypertensive SOD pressure greater than 40 mm Hg (Figure 47-1). The data for establishing this normal pressure of less than 40 mm Hg are based on extremely limited data. Whether endoscopic retrograde cholangiopancreatography (ERCP) in patients with suspected SOD is performed for diagnostic SOM or therapeutic purposes, complication rates are high.

Once the diagnosis of SOD is made, endoscopic sphincterotomy is the treatment of choice as it is believed to decrease the risk of recurrent pancreatitis. The Geenen-Hogan (Milwaukee) criteria was devised to predict the overall probability of response to biliary sphincterotomy taking into account the presence of abnormal liver chemistries and dilated bile ducts. On the basis of this type I, patients with pain and both abnormalities are definitely recommended to have sphincterotomy as they have high response rates ranging from 90% to 100% regardless of SOM. Along this stratification, type II patients have either abnormal liver chemistry or dilated bile ducts. If SOM is abnormal in type II patients, they will have a response rate to sphincterotomy of 60% to 91% and thus this would be a reasonable course of action. On the contrary, type III patients do not have objective biliary abnormalities and even if they have abnormal SOM they have poor response rates of 6% to 58%, making sphincterotomy of questionable benefit.

Patients with SOD are at a high risk for developing post-ERCP pancreatitis. Pancreatic stent placement decreases the risk of post-ERCP pancreatitis in high-risk patients. Pancreatic duct stenting has become a common practice during ERCP in patients with SOD who undergo sphincterotomy. Pancreatic stenting is effective presumably because it prevents cannulation-induced edema that can lead to ductal obstruction. Pancreatic sphincter hypertension is a significant risk factor for post-ERCP pancreatitis, which may explain the high risk of pancreatitis in SOD patients. There is prolonged alleviation of ductal obstruction when pancreatic stents are placed. Typically, 3 to 5 French unflanged pancreatic stents are used in patients with SOD. Thirteen trials (6 prospective, randomized controlled trials and 7 case-control trials) have been published evaluating the role of pancreatic stent placement in the prevention of post-ERCP pancreatitis. In all of the reported studies, which cumulatively include 1500 high-risk patients undergoing ERCP, only 1 patient developed severe pancreatitis after a pancreatic duct stent had been placed.

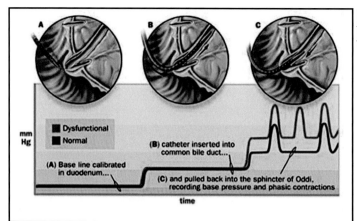

Figure 47-1. Method of performing sphincter of Oddi dysfunction manometry.

In summary, in a patient with recurrent pancreatitis or recurrent biliary-type pain found to have abnormal liver function tests and a dilated CBD not explained by tumor or stones, SOD (type I) is a reasonable diagnosis. Endoscopic sphincterotomy is the standard of care for treating these patients. In a patient with only similar symptoms, but only has abnormal liver function tests **or** a dilated CBD (type II), SOM may be needed prior to endoscopic sphincterotomy. The patient without abnormal liver function tests and/or a dilated CBD who has only pain, or even recurrent pancreatitis, will not likely benefit. In these patients, SOM has not been established as being useful in establishing the diagnosis. Consideration to limited but acceptable care for biliary-type irritable bowel syndrome is recommended. If endoscopic sphincterotomy for suspected SOD occurs, a pancreatic duct stent should be used to decrease the risk of severe acute pancreatitis.

Bibliography

Elta G. Sphincter of Oddi dysfunction and bile duct microlithiasis in acute idiopathic pancreatitis. *World J Gastroenterol.* 2008;14:1023-1026.

Freeman ML, Gill M, Overby C, Cen YY. Predictors of outcomes after biliary and pancreatic sphincterotomy for sphincter of oddi dysfunction. *J Clin Gastroenterol.* 2007;41:94-102.

Hogan WJ, Sherman S, Pasricha P, Carr-Locke D. Sphincter of Oddi manometry. *Gastrointest Endosc.* 1997;45:342-348.

Steinberg WM. Controversies in clinical pancreatology: should the sphincter of Oddi be measured in patients with idiopathic recurrent acute pancreatitis, and should sphincterotomy be performed if the pressure is high? *Pancreas.* 2003;27:118-121.

Wehrmann T, Wiemer K, Lembcke B, Caspary WF, Jung M. Do patients with sphincter of Oddi dysfunction benefit from endoscopic sphincterotomy? A 5-year prospective trial. *Eur J Gastroenterol Hepatol.* 1996;8:251-256.

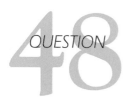
WHEN SHOULD A PANCREATIC DUCT STENT BE USED?

Ian Wall, DO and Robin Baradarian, MD, FACG

Flow of pancreatic juices can be impeded through a variety of changes within the duct itself or in the pancreatic portion of the sphincter of Oddi (SOD). This impedance can lead to intraductal hypertension and result in pain or pancreatic inflammation depending on the etiology and its acuity of onset. The etiology of impedance to ductal flow of pancreatic juices can broadly be divided into pancreatic duct obstruction and duct interruption. The primary goal of pancreatic duct stenting, regardless of the disease process, is to restore appropriate flow of pancreatic juices through the pancreatic duct into the duodenum.

Prophylaxis of Post-Endoscopic Retrograde Cholangiopancreatography Pancreatitis

Prophylactic placement of a pancreatic stent to prevent severe post-endoscopic retrograde cholangiopancreatography (ERCP) pancreatitis has become the standard of care in select patients. The value of prophylactic pancreatic stenting is realized in patients who are at a higher risk for post-ERCP pancreatitis. The established risk factors for post-ERCP pancreatitis are female sex, younger age, suspected SOD, prior episodes of post-ERCP pancreatitis, pancreatic duct injection, pancreatic sphincterotomy, balloon dilatation of an intact biliary sphincter, difficult cannulation, ampullectomy, and pre-cut sphincterotomy. These factors are additive when determining risk (Table 48-1). Typically, 3 to 5 French gauge, unflanged, plastic stents are used to provide the desired alleviation of ductal obstruction (Figure 48-1). In all of the reported studies, which cumulatively include 1500 high-risk patients undergoing ERCP, only 1 patient developed severe pancreatitis after a pancreatic duct stent had been placed.[1] A meta-analysis published in 2004 by Singh et al[2]

Table 48-1

Procedures in Which Placement of Pancreatic Duct Stent Should Be Considered

- Treatment of sphincter of Oddi dysfunction type I
- Prior history of post-endoscopic retrograde cholangiopancreatography pancreatitis
- Multiple pancreatic duct injections
- Difficult cannulation
- Pancreatic sphincterotomy
- Pre-cut access
- Balloon dilatation
- Ampullectomy

---

evaluating 5 prospective trials including 483 patients, showed a 3-fold reduction in the incidence of post-ERCP pancreatitis in patients with pancreatic duct stents vs no stent (15.5% vs 5.8%, p=0.001, OR 3.2, 95% CI [1.6, 6.4]). Similarly, a 2007 meta-analysis published by Andriulli et al[3] that evaluated 4 randomized, prospective trials including 268 patients, showed a 2-fold drop in the incidence of post-ERCP pancreatitis (24.1% vs 12%, p=0.009, OR 0.44, 95% CI [0.24, 0.81]). In a large, retrospective review of 2283 patients having a total of 2447 ERCPs, 3 French unflanged stents were more effective in reducing the incidence of post-ERCP pancreatitis (p=0.0043), more likely to pass spontaneously (p=0.0001), and less likely to cause ductal changes (24% vs 80%) when compared to larger 4, 5, or 6 French stents.[4] Prophylactic stent placement is a cost-effective strategy for the prevention of post-ERCP pancreatitis for high-risk patients.

Chronic Pancreatitis

Chronic pancreatitis through progressive fibrosis leads to pancreatic ductal strictures and ultimately obstruction of the pancreatic duct with subsequent increased pancreatic ductal pressures resulting in characteristic pain. Patients with a single major pancreatic duct stricture in the head of the pancreas are the best candidates for ductal stenting. Ideally, a large bore (10 French) stent is advanced past the stricture and may require dilatation prior to successful insertion. A recent review reported pain relief with 52% to 95% of patients over a period of 72 months.[5] Several controversial aspects remain with regards to pancreatic duct stenting for chronic pancreatitis including the need for stent exchange and its effectiveness compared with surgical intervention. A pancreatic stent's life is finite and will ultimately require an exchange within 6 to 9 months, increasing the risk and cost of this approach. Instead of a scheduled exchange, some endoscopists are moving toward an approach of "on demand" stent exchange in response to clinical signs and symptoms that indicate the stent is no longer functional.[6] A recent small study that employed a multistent approach to ductal strictures has been shown to be effective in dilating strictures and providing long-term relief of obstruction following stent removal.[7] Despite these newer technical advances, the optimal number of stents and time left indwelling remains

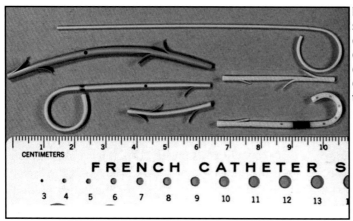

Figure 48-1. Pancreatic duct stents. Differences in size, diameter, and design are based on the underlying pancreatic disease to be treated, location of the disease, and diameter of the pancreatic duct.

to be determined. The second area of controversy concerns a comparison between an endoscopic vs surgical approach to ductal strictures. A head-to-head comparison of endoscopic vs surgical intervention (pancreaticojejunostomy) in chronic pancreatitis found more rapid and sustained pain relief in the surgical arm.[8] The ultimate role for pancreatic stenting and endoscopic treatment in general for chronic pancreatitis is constantly being redefined and remains controversial. The continuum ranges from definitive treatment for limited disease to a bridge to surgery for more extensive and complex disease.

Prophylaxis During Endoscopic Ampullectomy

Ampullectomy is a well-established technique to remove tumors that arise in the area of the major duodenal papilla. Post-procedure pancreatitis was frequently found as a result of procedure-related edema around the pancreatic duct outflow and resultant obstruction. A prospective randomized controlled trial by Harewood et al[9] confirmed the benefits of prophylactic pancreatic stent placement in patients undergoing ampullectomy to avoid post-procedure pancreatitis.

Endoscopic Management of Pancreas Divisum

Pancreas divisum is a common congenital defect of the pancreas and can result, in some people, in recurrent pancreatitis or chronic pain. Endoscopic therapy has been found to be most effective in patients with recurrent acute pancreatitis and progressively less effective with patients with chronic pancreatitis and those with chronic abdominal pain. The endoscopic procedure consists of minor papilla sphincterotomy and dorsal duct stenting. Controversy exists regarding how long the pancreatic duct stent should remain in place as several series have found changes within the duct including dilatation and stenosis following stent removal. These changes tend to improve with time but there is no evidence regarding long-term consequences. A prospective randomized blinded trial is needed to truly demonstrate if pancreatic duct stending in pancreas divisum is effective.

Pancreatic Duct Disruptions

Ductal interruption is the second broad category of patients who benefit from pancreatic ductal stenting to re-establish proper flow of pancreatic juices. The two major causes of pancreatic ductal interruption are trauma to the pancreas and pancreatic fluid collection formation with main pancreatic duct communication due to pancreactic inflammation. Pancreatic peritoneal fistulas leading to massive ascites and pancreatic pleural fistulas leading to massive pleural effusions are amenable to the placement of pancreatic duct stents bridging the area of disruption on ERCP. Typically, this intervention is successful in treating these disorders. Even if the stent cannot be placed beyond the area of disruption, shorter stents that simply open the pancreatic duct and pancreatic papilla to equalize pressures to the duodenum enhance drainage.

Drainage of Pancreatic Fluid Collections and Pseudocysts

Pancreatic fluid collections are the result of inflammation associated with chronic pancreatitis or following an episode of acute pancreatitis. In the patient with acute pancreatitis, Kozarek and colleagues[10] have been evaluating the role of early stent placement to prevent complications, organ failure, and pseudocysts. However, at this time, further study is needed. Most fluid collections resolve spontaneously and drainage is not needed. In patients with symptomatic pseudocysts, which typically develop after a month from the onset of acute pancreatitis or in the setting of chronic pancreatitis, endoscopic placement of a pancreatic stent can help resolution. It must be remembered that pancreatic stent placement for pseudocysts is reserved for patients who (1) do not have pancreatic necrosis (eg, debris in the cyst), (2) have a cyst that communicates, and (3) have a cyst that is symptomatic (eg, infection or pain or early satiety/weight loss). A large review of the endoscopic management of pancreatic fluid collections and pseudocysts found a high clinical success rate with collections drained by pancreatic duct stenting alone and pancreatic duct stenting combined with transmural drainage, 93% and 83%, respectively. Pancreatic duct drainage was achieved with stent placement past the area of interruption or directly into the fluid collection/pseudocyst. In summary, pancreatic duct stenting is indicated in (1) patients undergoing high-risk ERCP in order to prevent severe post-ERCP pancreatitis, (2) patients with pain from chronic pancreatitis who are suffering from pain and have a dominant stricture or stone, (3) patients who have ductal disruptions leading to pancreatic peritoneal fistulas or pancreatic pleural fistulas, and (4) for drainage procedures, such as pseudocysts that communicate with pancreatic duct. Further study is ongoing determining the role of pancreatic duct stenting in acute pancreatitis, but at this point in time, unless a patient has a smoldering and persisting form of pancreatitis with persistent duct leakage, a conservative approach should be taken.

References

1. Badalov N, Tenner S, Baillie J. The prevention, recognition and treatment of Post-ERCP Pancreatitis. *JOP.* 2009;10:83-97.
2. Singh P, Sivak MV, Agarwal D, et al. Prophylactic pancreatic stenting for prevention of post-ERCP acute pancreatitis: a meta-analysis of controlled trials. [abstract] *Gastrointest Endosc.* 2003;57:AB89.
3. Andriulli A, Forlano R, Napolitano G, et al. Pancreatic duct stents in the prophylaxis of pancreatic damage after endoscopic retrograde cholangiopancreatography: a systematic analysis of benefits and associated risks. *Digestion.* 2007;75:156-163.
4. Rashdan A, Fogel EL, McHenry L, Sherman S, Temkit M, Lehman GA. Improved stent characteristics for prophylaxis of post-ERCP pancreatitis. *Clinical Gastroenterology and Hepatology.* 2004;2:322-329.
5. Tringali A, Boskoski I, Costamagna G. The role of endoscopy in the therapy of chronic pancreatitis. *Best Pract Res Clin Gastroenterol.* 2008;22:145-165.
6. Wilcox CM, Varadarajulu S. Endoscopic therapy for chronic pancreatitis: an evidence based review. *Curr Gastroenterol Rep.* 2006;8:104-110.
7. Costamagna G, Bulajic M, Tringali A, et al. Multiple stenting of refractory pancreatic duct strictures in severe chronic pancreatitis: long-term results. *Endoscopy.* 2006;38:254-259.
8. Cahen DL, Gouma DJ, Nio Y, et al. Endoscopic versus surgical drainage of the pancreatic duct in chronic pancreatitis. *N Engl J Med.* 2007;356:676-684.
9. Harewood GC, Pochron NL, Gostout CJ. Prospectiv, randomized, controlled trial of prophylactic pancreatic stent placement for endoscopic snare excision of the duodenal ampulla. *Gastrointest Endosc.* 2005;62:367-370.
10. Kozarek RA. Endoscopic therapy of complete and partial pancreatic duct disruptions. *Gastrointest Endosc Clin N Am.* 1998;8:39-53.

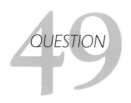
How Do I Evaluate for and Treat Patients With Autoimmune Pancreatitis?

Shishir K. Maithel, MD and Charles M. Vollmer, Jr, MD

Autoimmune pancreatitis (AIP) is a relatively rare disorder of the pancreas. Although initially described in elderly male patients, recently reported case series have shown the disorder to be quite heterogeneous. There appears to be an increased incidence in some regions around the world, particularly in Japan. It remains to be seen whether this represents merely an increased clinical awareness or due to an actual increased prevalence of the disease.

Although it has been described as a primary pancreatic disorder, it is often associated with other diseases of autoimmune etiology, such as sclerosing cholangitis, primary biliary cirrhosis, retroperitoneal fibrosis, inflammatory bowel disease, sarcoidosis, rheumatoid arthritis, and Sjogren's syndrome. The concurrent involvement of other autoimmune diseases suggests that AIP may be part of a larger syndrome complex rather than an isolated clinical entity.

The immunologic derangement that leads to AIP seems to involve both humoral and cellular components. An abnormality of the humoral immune system implies that a patient possesses autoantibodies to an endogenous antigen. Given the fact that AIP is often associated with other autoimmune phenomena, it appears that there may be a common antigen in the pancreas and other exocrine organs such as the salivary glands, biliary tract, and renal tubules that is recognized by autoantibodies.

The clinical symptoms of AIP are usually distinct from those of acute pancreatitis from other causes. Patients with AIP often have no, or only slight, discomfort in the mid-epigastrium or back. They can present, however, with symptoms of longer chronicity, which may consist of anorexia, steatorrhea, new onset diabetes, and weight loss. Often, patients only present with an incidental pancreatic mass or fullness that is discovered on axial imaging which raises the concern for malignancy (Figure 49-1). Due to the presence of a

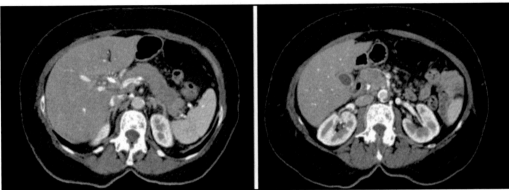

Figure 49-1. Computed tomography imaging of autoimmune pancreatitis that reveals characteristic fullness of the pancreas.

Table 49-1

Japan Pancreas Society Diagnostic Criteria for Autoimmune Pancreatitis (2002)

1. Pancreatic imaging shows diffuse enlargement of the pancreas with diffuse (>33%) narrowing of the main pancreatic duct with irregular walls
2. Abnormally elevated levels of serum gammaglobulin, and/or immunoglobulin G, or the presence of autoantibodies
3. Histopathology reveals lymphoplasmacytic infiltration and fibrotic changes of the pancreas

Diagnostic criteria for autoimmune pancreatitis (2002) as proposed by the Japan Pancreas Society. Criterion 1 must be present with criterion 2 and/or 3 to make the diagnosis of autoimmune pancreatitis.

---

concomitant biliary stricture, patients may present with new onset jaundice and the liver function enzyme profile will have a characteristic obstructive pattern. The serum amylase and lipase levels can be elevated as well. Radiographically, the presentation can vary from diffuse changes throughout the whole pancreas to minimal radiographic signs.

The diagnostic criteria for AIP are in evolution, partly because this is a relatively new clinical entity. The basis for making the diagnosis of AIP was first described by the Japan Pancreas Society[1] in 2002. The diagnosis rests on 3 criteria involving imaging, laboratory data, and histopathological findings, the details of which are outlined in Table 49-1. According to this framework, in order to make the diagnosis, criterion 1 must be present along with criterion 2 and/or 3. The hallmark finding on histopathologic analysis is the presence of lymphoplasmacytic sclerosing pancreatitis (LPSP), along with foci of fibrotic changes.

As the diagnosis of AIP has increased in incidence and gained recognition over the past few years, the limitations of the Japan Pancreas Society definition have become apparent. For example, some patients may not meet the radiologic criterion of diffuse pancreatic enlargement but still harbor the characteristic histopathologic changes. Recognizing the

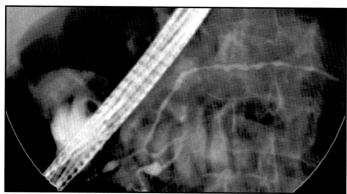

Figure 49-2. Endoscopic retrograde cholangiopancreatography showing diffuse narrowing of the main pancreatic duct consistent with the diagnosis of autoimmune pancreatitis. The duct became normal in appearance after a course of prednisone.

Table 49-2

Extended Diagnostic Criteria for Autoimmune Pancreatitis (Mayo Clinic)

Imaging	Satisfies Japan Pancreas Society criteria or presence of focal pancreatic mass/enlargement; focal pancreatic duct stricture; pancreatic atrophy; pancreatic calcification; or pancreatitis
Serology	Elevated serum immunoglobulin G4 level
Histology	At least 1 of the following: (1) periductal lymphoplasmacytic infiltrate with obliterative phlebitis and storiform fibrosis or (2) lymphoplasmacytic infiltrate with storiform fibrosis and abundant immunoglobulin G4-positive cells (≥10 cells/high power field)
Other organ involvement	Hilar/intrahepatic biliary strictures; persistent distal biliary stricture; parotid/lacrimal gland involvement; mediastinal lymphadenopathy; retroperitoneal fibrosis
Response to steroid therapy	Resolution or marked improvement of pancreatic/extrapancreatic manifestation with steroid therapy

existing shortcomings and the need for more inclusive criteria, the Mayo Clinic has developed expanded diagnostic criteria for AIP, which not only includes imaging, serology, and histology, but also 2 other categories of (1) other organ involvement and (2) response to steroid therapy. The details of these expanded criteria are outlined in Table 49-2. On the basis of their experience, they have defined 3 groups of patients that can be diagnosed with AIP: (1) those with characteristic histology (LPSP) and/or pancreatic immunoglobulin G4 (IgG4) immunostaining, (2) those who meet Japanese imaging criteria and also have elevated serum IgG4 levels, and (3) those whose pancreatic/extrapancreatic disease responds to steroid therapy in the setting of unexplained pancreatic disease and/or elevated serum IgG4 levels.

Magnetic resonance or endoscopic retrograde cholangiopancreatography may also reveal a characteristic narrowing of the pancreatic duct. This narrowing can be focal, segmental, or diffuse (Figure 49-2). At times, the common bile duct is involved resulting in dilatation of the common bile duct. In general, diagnostic imaging should be confirmed by either serologic or histologic analysis. Elevated levels of the specific subtype IgG4 are frequently associated with AIP, although this laboratory finding is not an absolute prerequisite for making the diagnosis. Elevated serum titers of antilactoferrin antibodies and/or anticarbonic anhydrase antibodies are also suggestive of AIP. Pathologic confirmation may be obtained by endoscopic ultrasound and fine needle aspiration. Some have suggested that a core biopsy could increase the accuracy of histologic analysis.

It is imperative, however, to understand that pancreatic cancer is much more common than AIP. Thus, patients with obstructive jaundice of evasive etiology should not be empirically started on high-dose steroid therapy unless actual diagnostic criteria are met for AIP. If an open pancreatic biopsy is required to make the correct diagnosis, then it should be performed. However, this approach should be limited to the few patients in which this diagnosis cannot be established by other accepted criteria.

The mainstay of therapy for AIP is systemic corticosteroids. The response rate is variable, but typically ranges in the order of 1 to 4 months. The usual regimen of prednisone therapy is to initiate therapy with high doses (eg, 40 mg/day) and then to institute a slow taper based on clinical response. The duration of therapy is variable, depending upon each patient's response to therapy. Some patients (approximately 25%) may relapse, thus requiring a second course of treatment, and an even smaller percentage of patients may require lifelong low-dose steroid therapy in order to maintain remission.

The long-term prognosis and clinical sequelae of AIP is currently undefined, mostly because this is a relatively newly recognized clinical entity. Most of the clinical changes associated with AIP, aside from established pancreatic fibrosis, are reversible with steroid therapy. Long-term prognosis may also be in part dependent on the severity of complications or manifestations of other associated autoimmune disease.

References

1. Japan Pancreas Society. Diagnostic criteria for autoimmune pancreatitis by the Japan Pancreas Society. *Journal of the Japan Pancreas Society*. 2002;17:585.

Bibliography

Chari ST, Smyrk TC, Levy MJ, et al. Diagnosis of autoimmune pancreatitis: the Mayo Clinic experience. *Clinical Gastroenterology and Hepatology*. 2006;4:1010.

Finkelberg DL, Sahani D, Vikhram D, Brugge WR. Autoimmune pancreatitis. *N Engl J Med*. 2006;355:2670-2676.

Okazaki K. Autoimmune pancreatitis: etiology, pathogenesis, clinical findings and treatment. The Japanese experience. *J Pancreas*. 2005;6(Suppl 1):89.

INDEX

acute cholecystitis, biliary colic, distinguishing, 12
acute gallstone pancreatitis, 33-35
acute pancreatitis, 1-65
advanced pancreatic cancer, 153-156
age as risk factor, 143
alcohol-induced injury to pancreas, 87-89
algorithm, diagnosing pancreatic cancer, 150
ampullectomy, 232
    endoscopic prophylaxis, 233
antibiotics, 15-19
ascites, pancreatic, with chronic pancreatitis, 98
atrophy of gland, 70
autoimmune pancreatitis, 91-96, 237-240
    computed tomography, 92
    diagnosis, 92
    endoscopic retrograde
      cholangiopancreatography, 93
    endoscopic ultrasound, 93-94
    HISORt criteria, 95
    histology, 94-95
    Japanese Pancreas Society criteria, 238
    labs, 92
    magnetic resonance imaging, 92

balloon dilatation, 232
Balthazar grading system, computed tomography, 14
bile duct stone evaluation, 183-186
biliary colic, acute cholecystitis, distinguishing, 12
biliary obstruction, with chronic pancreatitis, 98
biliary sludge, 50-51
biliary tract, 175-223

C-reactive protein, 7-9
    for determination of severity of pancreatitis, 8
calcifications, 70
Cambridge classification, 73
cancer, pancreatic
    advanced pancreatic cancer, 153-156
    age, 143
    chronic pancreatitis, 143-144
    diabetes mellitus, 144
    diet, 144
    familial pancreatic cancer, 145
    gender, 144
    nonpancreatic cancer syndromes, 145-146
    obesity, 145
    partial gastrectomy, 145
    risk factors, 143-146
    smoking, 145
    staging, 147-152
      alternative approach, 150
      determining resectability, 149
      diagnosing pancreatic cancer algorithm,
        150
      staging of pancreatic exocrine cancer,
        150-152
      traditional approach, 149
cannulation, 232
Caroli's disease, 203-208
causes of hypergastrinemia, 168
cholangiocarcinoma, 215-219
    cytologic diagnosis, 217
cholangiopancreatography, retrograde, 21-24, 93,
    183-186

cholangiopancreatoscopy, 177-181
cholangioscopes, 178
cholangitis, sclerosing
    endoscopic, 200
    management, 200
    medical, 200
    surgical management, 200
    transplantation, 200
cholecystectomy, 37-39, 41-43
cholecystitis, 12
    biliary colic, distinguishing, 12
choledochal cyst, 209-214
    classification of, 211
chronic diarrhea, 163-165
    VIPoma diagnosis, 163-165
chronic pancreatitis, 67-100, 143-144, 232-233
    alcohol-induced injury to pancreas, 87-89
    pseudoaneurysm, 100
    pseudocyst with, 98
classification of choledochal cysts, 211
classification of masses in pancreas, 172
clinical differences between cystic neoplasms of
    pancreas, 117
clinical response to therapy meta-analysis, 84
closed-loop intestinal obstruction, acute
    cholecystitis, distinguishing, 12
commercially available cholangioscopes, 178
common bile duct obstruction, 99
comparison of imaging methods for detection of
    cholangiocarcinoma, 217
complications of chronic pancreatitis, 97-100
computed tomography, 11-14, 71-72, 92
computed tomography grading system of Balthazar,
    14
criteria for autoimmune pancreatitis, Japanese
    Pancreas Society, 238
Crohn's disease, 59-61
current approaches to management of pain in
    chronic pancreatitis, 78
cyst fluid analysis, 105
cystic lesions, 101-139
    endoscopic therapy, 135-139
    endoscopic ultrasonographer, computed
        tomography-guided fine needle aspiration,
        119-121
    endoscopic ultrasound-guided fine needle
        aspiration, pancreatic cyst, amylase,
        111-113
    infected pseudocyst, 127-130
    pancreatic cyst, 131-134
    pseudocyst, 123-126
    serous cystadenoma, mucinous cystadenoma,
        distinguished, 115-118
    tail of pancreas

cystic lesion, 107-109
    fluid-filled cyst, 103-105
cytologic diagnosis, 217
    cholangiocarcinoma, 217
cytologic diagnosis of cholangiocarcinoma, 217

definition of TNM, 152
determining resectability, 149
diabetes mellitus, 144
diagnosing algorithm, 150
    pancreatic cancer, 150
diagnosing pancreatic cancer algorithm, 150
diagnosis of chronic pancreatitis, 69-75
diarrhea, VIPoma diagnosis, 163-165
diet, 144
differences in cyst fluid analysis of pancreatic cystic
    neoplasms, 118
dilated pancreatic ducts, 70
discussion with patient, 187-189
dissecting aortic aneurysm, acute cholecystitis,
    distinguishing, 12
"double duct sign," endoscopic retrograde
    cholangiopancreatography, 183-186
drainage, pancreatic fluid, pseudocysts, 234
duct disruptions, 234
duct stent, 231-235
    chronic pancreatitis, 232-233
    drainage, pancreatic fluid collections,
        pseudocysts, 234
    endoscopic ampullectomy, prophylaxis during,
        233
    pancreas divisum, endoscopic management,
        233
    pancreatic duct disruptions, 234
duct stones, 70
duodenal obstruction, 99

echotexture, 70
ectopic pregnancy, acute cholecystitis,
    distinguishing, 12
endoscopic ampullectomy, 233
    prophylaxis, 233
endoscopic approaches to pain, 79-80
endoscopic management, 79-80, 233
    pancreas divisum, 233
endoscopic prophylaxis, 233
endoscopic retrograde cholangiopancreatography,
    72-74, 93, 183-186, 191-195, 221-223
    acute gallstone pancreatitis, 33-35
    degree of difficulty grades, 223
    discussion with patient, 187-189
endoscopic therapy, 135-139
    organized necrosis, 135-139
    pseudocyst, 135-139

endoscopic ultrasonographer, computed tomography-guided fine needle aspiration, 119-121

endoscopic ultrasound, 74-75, 93-94

endoscopic ultrasound-guided fine needle aspiration, pancreatic cyst, amylase, 111-113

exocrine cancer, pancreatic, staging, 150-152

exocrine pancreatic cancer, staging, 150-152

extended diagnostic criteria for autoimmune pancreatitis, 239

factors increasing risk of post-endoscopic retrograde cholangiopancreatography pancreatitis, 22

familial pancreatic cancer, 145

fine needle aspiration, endoscopic ultrasound-guided, 111-113

flat plate of abdomen, 71

fluid, pancreatic, drainage, pseudocysts, 234

fluid analysis of pancreatic cystic neoplasms, differences in, 118

fluid during management of pancreatitis, 3-6

fluid-filled cyst, 103-105

gallstone pancreatitis, 33-35, 48, 191-195
    cholecystectomy, 37-39
    endoscopic retrograde cholangiopancreatography, 191-195
    magnetic resonance cholangiopancreatography, 191-195

gallstones, 29-31, 48

gas-producing organisms in pancreas, 48

gastrectomy, partial, 145

gastric outlet obstruction, with chronic pancreatitis, 98

gastrinoma evaluation, 167-169

gender, as risk factor, 144

genetic factors, 52

grading system, Balthazar, computed tomography, 14

grading system for major complications of endoscopic retrograde cholangiopancreatography and endoscopic sphincterotomy, 188

HISORt criteria, 95
    autoimmune pancreatitis, 95

HISORt criteria for autoimmune pancreatitis, 95

histology, 94-95

hypergastrinemia, causes of, 168

hypertriglyceridemia causing acute pancreatitis, 55-57

idiopathic pancreatitis, prior to establishing diagnosis, 50

imaging tests used in diagnosis of chronic pancreatitis, 70

indicators, pancreatic cancer risk
    age, 143
    chronic pancreatitis, 143-144
    diabetes mellitus, 144
    diet, 144
    familial pancreatic cancer, 145
    gender, 144
    nonpancreatic cancer syndromes, 145-146
    obesity, 145
    partial gastrectomy, 145
    smoking, 145

infarction, acute cholecystitis, distinguishing, 12

infected necrosis, 48

infected pseudocyst, 127-130

inferior wall myocardial infarction, acute cholecystitis, distinguishing, 12

Japanese Pancreas Society, criteria for autoimmune pancreatitis, 95, 238

lesions, cystic pancreatic, 101-139
    endoscopic therapy, 135-139
    endoscopic ultrasonographer, 119-121
    fine needle aspiration, 111-113
    infected pseudocyst, 127-130
    mucinous cystadenoma, 115-118
    pancreatic cyst, 131-134
    pseudocyst, 123-126
    serous cystadenoma, 115-118
    tail of pancreas
        cystic lesion, 107-109
        fluid-filled cyst, 103-105

Ludwig staging system, primary sclerosing cholangitis, 199

magnetic resonance cholangiopancreatography, 183-186, 191-195

margins of gland, 70

markers for pancreatic cancer risk
    age, 143
    chronic pancreatitis, 143-144
    diabetes mellitus, 144
    diet, 144
    familial pancreatic cancer, 145
    gender, 144
    nonpancreatic cancer syndromes, 145-146
    obesity, 145
    partial gastrectomy, 145
    smoking, 145

masses mimicking pancreatic cancer, 171-174

Mayo Clinic, extended diagnostic criteria for autoimmune pancreatitis, 239

medical treatment for pain, 78-79
mesenteric ischemia, infarction, acute cholecystitis, distinguishing, 12
meta-analysis therapy, clinical response, 84
microlithiasis, 42, 50-51
mucinous cystadenoma, serous cystadenoma, distinguished, 115-118
multisystem organ failure, progression of, 48

necrosis-worsening organ failure, 48
neoplasms, pancreatic, 141-174
    advanced pancreatic cancer, 153-156
    age, 143
    chronic pancreatitis, 143-144
    diabetes mellitus, 144
    diagnosing algorithm, 150
    diet, 144
    familial pancreatic cancer, 145
    gender, 144
    masses mimicking pancreatic cancer, 171-174
    nonpancreatic cancer syndromes, 145-146
    obesity, 145
    pancreatic cancer, 143-146
    partial gastrectomy, 145
    race, 144
    risk factors, 143-146
    smoking, 145
    staging, 147-152
        alternative approach, 150
        determining resectability, 149
        diagnosing pancreatic cancer algorithm, 150
        traditional approach, 149
nonpancreatic cancer syndromes, 145-146
nutrition, 25-28

obesity, 145
omeprazole, gastrinoma evaluation, 167-169
organ failure, progression of multisystem, 48
organized necrosis, 135-139
    endoscopic therapy, 135-139

pain, 77-81
    endoscopic approaches, 79-80
    medical treatment, 78-79
    surgical approaches, 80-81
pancreas divisum, 52, 233
    endoscopic management, 233
pancreatic adenocarcinoma, with chronic pancreatitis, 98
pancreatic ascites, 99
    with chronic pancreatitis, 98
pancreatic cancer, 141-156
    advanced pancreatic cancer, 153-156

age, 143
chronic pancreatitis, 143-144
diabetes mellitus, 144
diagnosing algorithm, 150
diet, 144
familial pancreatic cancer, 145
gender, 144
masses mimicking pancreatic cancer, 171-174
nonpancreatic cancer syndromes, 145-146
obesity, 145
partial gastrectomy, 145
race, 144
risk factors, 143-146
smoking, 145
staging, 147-152
    alternative approach, 150
    determining resectability, 149
    diagnosing pancreatic cancer algorithm, 150
    traditional approach, 149
pancreatic cyst, 131-134
pancreatic duct disruptions, 234
pancreatic duct stent, 231-235
    chronic pancreatitis, 232-233
    disruptions, 234
    drainage, pancreatic fluid collections, pseudocysts, 234
    endoscopic ampullectomy, prophylaxis during, 233
    pancreas divisum, endoscopic management, 233
pancreatic ductal stones, 70
pancreatic enzymes to treat pain, 83-85
pancreatic exocrine cancer, staging, 150-152
pancreatic fluid
    drainage, pseudocysts, 234
    pseudocysts, 234
pancreatic neoplasms, 157-174
    chronic diarrhea, VIPoma diagnosis, 163-165
    recurrent hypoglycemia, insulinoma evaluation, 159-161
    reflux esophagitis, with omeprazole, gastrinoma evaluation, 167-169
    VIPoma diagnosis, 163-165
pancreatic sphincterotomy, 232
pancreatitis, 1-65
pancreatoscopy findings in normal, diseased states of pancreas, 180
parenchyma, 70
partial gastrectomy, 145
patient, discussion with, 187-189
perforated hollow viscus, acute cholecystitis, distinguishing, 12
placement of pancreatic duct stent, procedures, 232

pleural effusion, 98-99
post-endoscopic retrograde
    cholangiopancreatography pancreatitis, 21-24
post-procedure pancreatitis, 187-189
    endoscopic retrograde
        cholangiopancreatography, 187-189
pregnancy, ectopic, acute cholecystitis,
    distinguishing, 12
primary sclerosing cholangitis, 197-201
    endoscopy, 200
    management, 200
    medical management, 200
    surgical management, 200
    transplantation, 200
prior to establishing diagnosis of idiopathic
    pancreatitis, 50
progression of multisystem organ failure, 48
prophylaxis, during endoscopic ampullectomy, 233
pseudoaneurysm, 48, 100
pseudocyst, 97-98, 123-126, 135-139, 234
    endoscopic therapy, 135-139
    with chronic pancreatitis, 98

race as risk factor, 144
randomized placebo-controlled studies evaluating
    intravenous antibiotic prophylaxis of acute
    necrotizing pancreatitis, 18
randomized trials comparing urgent endoscopic
    retrograde cholangiopancreatography to
    medical therapy, 34
recurrent, unexplained acute pancreatitis, 49-54
recurrent hypoglycemia, insulinoma evaluation,
    159-161
reflux esophagitis, with omeprazole, gastrinoma
    evaluation, 167-169
resectability, determination of, 149
retrograde cholangiopancreatography, 21-24, 93,
    183-186
risk factors, pancreatic cancer, 143-146
    age, 143
    chronic pancreatitis, 143-144
    diabetes mellitus, 144
    diet, 144
    familial pancreatic cancer, 145
    gender, 144
    nonpancreatic cancer syndromes, 145-146
    obesity, 145
    partial gastrectomy, 145
    smoking, 145

sclerosing cholangitis, 197-201
    endoscopic, 200
    management, 200
    medical, 200
    surgical management, 200

transplantation, 200
section chronic pancreatitis, 67-100
sepsis, failure to resolve with antibiotics, 48
serous cystadenoma, mucinous cystadenoma,
    distinguished, 115-118
6-mercaptopurine, azathioprine, case reports, 60
sludge, biliary, 50-51
smoking as risk factor, 145
sphincter of Oddi, 227-229
    classification of dysfunction, 51
    dysfunction of, 51
    type I dysfunction, 232
splenic vein thrombosis, 100
    with chronic pancreatitis, 98
staging pancreatic cancer, 147-152
    alternative approach, 150
    determining resectability, 149
    diagnosing pancreatic cancer algorithm, 150
    staging of pancreatic exocrine cancer, 150-152
    traditional approach, 149
stent, pancreatic duct, 231-235
    chronic pancreatitis, 232-233
    drainage, pancreatic fluid collections,
        pseudocysts, 234
    endoscopic ampullectomy, prophylaxis during,
        233
    pancreas divisum, endoscopic management,
        233
    pancreatic duct disruptions, 234
sterile necrosis-worsening organ failure, 48
stones, ductal, 70
summary of case reports of azathioprine, 6-
    mercaptopurine causing acute pancreatitis with
    rechallenge, 60
summary of idiopathic acute recurrent pancreatitis
    additional work-up, 53
surgical approaches to pain, 80-81

tail of pancreas
    cystic lesion, 107-109
    fluid-filled cyst, 103-105
therapy meta-analysis, clinical response to, 84
thrombosis, splenic vein, 100
    computed tomography, 63-65
tissue diagnosis of cholangiocarcinoma, 217
TNM, defined, 152
transplantation, 200
type I dysfunction of sphincter of Oddi, 232

ultrasonographer, endoscopic, 119-121
ultrasound
    abdominal, 71
    endoscopic, 93-94

VIPoma diagnosis, 163-165

Printed in the United States
by Baker & Taylor Publisher Services